Gastrointestinal Motility and Neurogastroenterology

Guest Editor

RICHARD W. MCCALLUM, MD,
FACP, FACG

GASTROINTESTINAL ENDOSCOPY CLINICS OF NORTH AMERICA

www.giendo.theclinics.com

Consulting Editor
CHARLES J. LIGHTDALE, MD

January 2009 • Volume 19 • Number 1

SAUNDERS an imprint of ELSEVIER, Inc.

W.B. SAUNDERS COMPANY
A Division of Elsevier Inc.

1600 John F. Kennedy Blvd. ● Suite 1800 ● Philadelphia, Pennsylvania 19103-2899

http://www.giendo.theclinics.com

GASTROINTESTINAL ENDOSCOPY CLINICS OF NORTH AMERICA Volume 19, Number 1
January 2009 ISSN 1052-5157, ISBN-13: 978-1-4377-0478-5, ISBN-10: 1-4377-0478-6

Editor: Kerry Holland

Gastrointestinal Endoscopy Clinics of North America (ISSN 1052-5157) is published quarterly by Elsevier Inc., 360 Park Avenue South, New York, NY 10010-1710. Months of issue are January, April, July, and October. Business and Editorial Offices: 1600 John F. Kennedy Blvd., Suite 1800, Philadelphia, PA, 19103-2899. Customer Service Office: 6277 Sea Harbor Drive, Orlando, FL 32887-4800. Periodicals postage paid at New York, NY and additional mailing offices. Subscription prices are $259.00 per year of US individuals $386.00 per year for US institutions, $133.00 per year for US students and residents, $286.00 per year for Canadian individuals, $471.00 per year for Canadian institutions, $362.00 per year for international individuals, $471.00 per year for international institutions, and $185.00 per year for Canadian and foreign students/residents. To receive student/resident rate, orders must be accompanied by name of affiliated institution, date of term, and the *signature* of program/residency coordinator on institution letterhead. Orders will be billed at individual rate until proof of status is received. Foreign air speed delivery is included in all *Clinics* subscription prices. All prices are subject to change without notice. **POSTMASTER:** Send address change to *Gastrointestinal Endoscopy Clinics of North America*, Elsevier Periodicals Customer Service, 11830 Westline Industrial Drive, St. Louis, MO 63146. **Customer Service: 1-800-654-2452 (US). From outside the United States, call 1-314-453-7041. Fax: 1-314-453-5170. E-mail: JournalsCustomerService-usa@elsevier.com (for print support) or JournalsOnline Support-usa@elsevier.com (for online support).**

Reprints. For copies of 100 or more, of articles in this publication, please contact the Commercial Reprints Department, Elsevier Inc., 360 Park Avenue South, New York, NY 10010-1710. Tel. (212) 633-3812; Fax: (212) 482-1935; email: reprints@elsevier.com.

Gastrointestinal Endoscopy Clinics of North America is covered in *Excerpta Medica, MEDLINE/PubMed (Index Medicus), and MEDLINE/MEDLARS.*

Printed and bound by CPI Group (UK) Ltd, Croydon, CR0 4YY

Transferred to Digital Print 2011

Contributors

CONSULTING EDITOR

CHARLES J. LIGHTDALE, MD
Professor, Department of Medicine, Columbia University Medical Center, New York, New York

GUEST EDITOR

RICHARD W. McCALLUM, MD, FACP, FACG
Professor, Department of Medicine, Director, Center for GI Nerve & Muscle Function, Division of GI Motility, Kansas University Medical Center, Kansas City, Kansas

AUTHORS

IAN M. CARROLL, PhD
Division of Gastroenterology and Hepatology, University of North Carolina at Chapel Hill School of Medicine, Chapel Hill, North Carolina

DOUGLAS A. DROSSMAN, MD
Professor of Medicine and Psychiatry, C-Director UNC Center for Functional GI and Motility Disorders, University of North Carolina, Chapel Hill, North Carolina

RONNIE FASS, MD
Professor of Medicine, and Head, Neuroenteric Clinical Research Group, Section of Gastroenterology, Department of Medicine, Southern Arizona VA Health Care System and University of Arizona Health Sciences Center, Tucson, Arizona

MADHUSUDAN GROVER, MD
Resident Physician, Division of Internal Medicine, Michigan State University, East Lansing, Michigan

REZA A. HEJAZI, MD
Research Scholar, Department of Medicine, Center for GI Nerve & Muscle Function, Division of GI Motility, Kansas University Medical Center, Kansas City, Kansas

SHIH-KUANG S. HONG, MD
Department of Gastroenterology and Hepatology, Clinical Research and Center for Swallowing and Esophageal Disorders, Vanderbilt University Medical Center, Nashville, Tennessee

RICHARD W. McCALLUM, MD
Professor, Department of Medicine, Director, Center for GI Nerve & Muscle Function, Division of GI Motility, Kansas University Medical Center, Kansas City, Kansas

WILLIAM C. ORR, PhD
Clinical Professor of Medicine, Lynn Health Science Institute, University of Oklahoma Health Sciences Center, Oklahoma City, Oklahoma

HENRY P. PARKMAN, MD
Professor of Medicine, Gastroenterology Section, Department of Medicine, Temple University School of Medicine, Philadelphia, Pennsylvania

RODRIGO A. PINTO, MD
Research Fellow, Department of Colorectal Surgery, Cleveland Clinic Florida, Weston, Florida

SATISH S.C. RAO, MD, PhD, FRCP (Lon)
Professor of Medicine, Director, Neurogastroenterology and Gastrointestinal Motility, Division of Gastroenterology & Hepatology, Department of Internal Medicine, University of Iowa Carver College of Medicine; and Division of Gastroenterology, University of Iowa Hospitals and Clinics, Iowa City, Iowa

YEHUDA RINGEL, MD
Associate Professor of Medicine, Division of Gastroenterology and Hepatology, University of North Carolina at Chapel Hill School of Medicine, Chapel Hill, North Carolina

DANA R. SANDS, MD, FACS, FASCRS
Director, Colorectal Physiology Center, Staff Surgeon, Department of Colorectal Surgery, Cleveland Clinic Florida, Weston; Voluntary Assistant Professor, University of Miami, Miami, Florida

C. DANIEL SMITH, MD
Professor and Chair, Department of Surgery, Mayo Clinic, Jacksonville, Florida

JEREMY STAPLETON, DO
Fellow in Training, Division of Gastroenterology/Hepatology, University of Louisville School of Medicine, Louisville, Kentucky

JOHN M. WO, MD
Associate Professor, Department of Medicine, Division of Gastroenterology/Hepatology, University of Louisville School of Medicine, Louisville, Kentucky

MICHAEL F. VAEZI, MD, PhD, MSc (Epi)
Professor of Medicine, Clinical Director, Department of Gastroenterology and Hepatology, and Director, Clinical Research and Center for Swallowing and Esophageal Disorders, Vanderbilt University Medical Center, Nashville, Tennessee

Contents

> Diagnostic testing for GERD has evolved to include multi esophageal sites (distal, proximal and hypopharyngeal monitoring), wireless pH, and oropharyngeal devices. The versatility of the devices has increased our ability to better understand the role of acid reflux in various disorders involving reflux of acid. Wireless pH monitoring improves patient comfort and allows monitoring for gastroesophageal reflux events over several days. Ambulatory MII-pH monitoring is another exciting diagnostic tool, which is capable of detecting more than one type of reflux and achieves higher sensitivity and specificity to detect GERD than endoscopy or pH-metry. It is useful in patients with either typical or atypical reflux symptoms who are refractory to proton pump inhibitor (PPI) therapy. In this setting, MII-pH can be performed on PPI therapy to assess the efficacy of PPIs and the role of nonacid or acid reflux in persistent symptoms.

> Functional heartburn is considered one of the most common functional esophageal disorders. The disorder is more common in young women and is associated with other functional bowel disorders and sychological co-morbidity, primarily somatization. The etiology of functional heartburn remains unknown. Most patients, however, demonstrate esophageal hypersensitivity. Functional heartburn has been identified as the main cause for proton pump inhibitor (PPI) failure in patients with heartburn. Treatment is still a challenge, and patients should be started with PPI treatment. In non-responders, escalation of the PPI dose could be attempted and, if unsuccessful, pain modulators should be prescribed.

> Gastroesophageal reflux is a very common condition, and surgery remains a reasonable options in select patients. Successful surgical care for GERD

depends on proper patient selection, workup and operative technique. This manuscript reviews surgical care for GERD.

Henry P. Parkman

Gastric and small-bowel dysfunction can include gastroparesis, functional dyspepsia, and even irritable bowel syndrome. Patients with symptoms suggesting these disorders are commonly encountered by a variety of physicians, especially gastroenterologists. In most patients, the physical examination and upper endoscopy are normal, and thus symptoms are suggested to be from a motility disorder or a functional gastrointestinal disorder. Further evaluation directed at evaluating the stomach and small-bowel motility may help the clinician to arrive at a correct diagnosis enabling proper treatment of the patient. This article covers several tests that are used to evaluate gastric and small-bowel motility in patients, either in clinical evaluation or in clinical research.

Jeremy Stapleton and John M. Wo

Gastroparesis is a symptomatic chronic disorder characterized by delayed gastric emptying without a mechanical obstruction. Gastroparesis is most often associated with diabetes, gastric surgery, and systemic disorders affecting the neuromuscular control of the stomach. However, no underlying etiology can be found in up to 40% of patients, a condition referred to as idiopathic gastroparesis. Due to the numerous potential etiologies and the highly variable clinical manifestations, the management of gastroparesis is particularly challenging. The purpose of this review is to provide an update on the use of antiemetics, prokinetics, and tricyclics for the treatment for nausea and vomiting associated with gastroparesis.

Reza A. Hejazi and Richard W. McCallum

Refractory gastroparesis is a challenging disorder for gastroenterologists, internists, surgeons, and all health care professionals involved in the care of these patients. It should be managed by a stepwise algorithm beginning with dietary modifications, then prokinetic and antiemetic medications, measures to control pain and address psychological issues, and endoscopic or surgical options in selected patients, including placement of feeding jejunostomy tubes.

Rodrigo A. Pinto and Dana R. Sands

Fecal continence is a complex bodily function, which requires the interplay of sensation, rectal capacity, and anal neuromuscular function. Fecal incontinence affects approximately 2% of the population and has a prevalence of 15% in elderly patients. Constipation is one of the most common gastrointestinal disorders. The variety of symptoms and risk factors suggest a multifactorial origin. Before any invasive intervention, the surgeon should have a thorough understanding of the etiology of these conditions. Appropriate medical management can improve symptoms in the majority of patients. Surgery is indicated when all medical possibilities are exhausted. This review discusses the most used surgical procedures emphasizing the latest experiences. Sacral nerve stimulation (SNS) is a promising option for patients with fecal incontinence and constipation. The procedure affords patients improved continence and quality of life. The mechanism of action is still poorly understood. This treatment has been used before in other more invasive surgical procedures or even after their failure to improve patients' symptoms and avoid a definitive stoma.

This article focuses on the colonic and anorectal motility disturbances that are associated with chronic constipation and their management. Functional chronic constipation consists of three overlapping subtypes: slow transit constipation, dyssynergic defecation, and irritable bowel syndrome with constipation. The Rome criteria may serve as a useful guide for making a clinical diagnosis of functional constipation. Today, an evidence-based approach can be used to treat patients with chronic constipation. The availability of specific drugs for the treatment of chronic constipation, such as tegaserod and lubiprostone, has enhanced the therapeutic armamentarium for managing these patients. Randomized controlled trials have also established the efficacy of biofeedback therapy in the treatment of dyssynergic defecation.

Functional gastrointestinal disorders (FGIDs) are highly prevalent in Western countries yet no single mechanism or etiological agent that initiates IBS has been identified. Current research has implicated the intestinal microbiota with FGIDs. This article reviews the available literature/data regarding the intestinal microbiota and FGIDS. The possible relationships between the intestinal microbiota and the intestinal function and functional bowel symptoms are discussed.

Functional gastrointestinal disorders (FGIDs) are commonly seen gastrointestinal (GI) conditions that are diagnosed using established symptom-based criteria. These disorders that typically defy traditional diagnostic methods based on structural abnormalities have intrigued researchers for several decades. This has led to the emergence of the current discipline of neurogastroenterology or the study of the "brain-gut axis," which is based on dysregulation of neuroenteric pathways as a key pathophysiologic feature of the FGIDs. Psychopharmacologic and behavioral treatments can influence the dysregulation of these pathways, especially at the severe end of the spectrum, and improve the clinical manifestations of these conditions, visceral discomfort or pain and bowel dysfunction. Their actions are mostly at spinal and supraspinal levels with some direct benefits at the level of the gut. Improvements in coping, global distress, and overall quality of life (QOL) have been shown more consistently with these treatments compared with improvement in GI symptoms. A successful approach to patients with these treatments requires a good physician–patient relationship. Strategizing treatments with these modalities is based on recognition of their dual effects on brain and gut, understanding the nature and severity of the GI symptoms and their psychosocial concomitants, and applying them within the context of the patient's understanding of their value.

Abnormalities of gastrointestinal (GI) motor function contribute directly or indirectly to a number of common clinical problems and account for significant health care–related expenditure. Proper evaluation of patients who have suspected GI motility disorders is important to ensure a correct diagnosis and to embark on an appropriate plan of treatment. The GI motility laboratory serves as an important area for patient evaluation in gastroenterology and is an essential element in any comprehensive digestive disease program. This article addresses important concepts in setting up and running an efficient and practical GI motility laboratory.

FORTHCOMING ISSUES

April 2009
Endoscopic Imaging
Grace Elta, MD, and Kenneth Wang, MD, *Guest Editors*

July 2009
Enteroscopy
David R. Cave, MD, *Guest Editor*

RECENT ISSUES

October 2008
Endoscopic Sedation: Preparing for the Future
Lawrence B. Cohen, MD,
and James Aisenberg, MD, *Guest Editors*

July 2008
Gastrointestinal Cancer and the Endoscopist: A Brave New World of Imaging and Treatment
Richard C. Boland, MD,
Pankaj Jay, Pasricha, MD,
and Kentaro Sugano, MD, PhD,
Guest Editors

April 2008
Natural Orifice Translumenal Endoscopic Surgery
Anthony N. Kalloo, MD, *Guest Editor*

RELATED INTEREST

Gastroenterology Clinics of North America, September 2007 (Vol. 36, Number 3)
Gastrointestinal Motility Disorders
Hanry Parkman, MD, *Guest Editor*

THE CLINICS ARE NOW AVAILABLE ONLINE!

Access your subscription at:
www.theclinics.com

Foreword

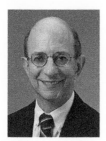

Charles J. Lightdale, MD
Consulting Editor

From the esophagus to the colon, gastrointestinal (GI) endoscopists have long been able to observe the movements of the GI tract but have often left the more detailed and quantitative analysis of GI motility to colleagues who have special interests in the management of "functional" disorders and a few specific diseases. Recent years, however, have seen major advances in the capability to analyze, understand, and treat GI motility disorders, with great potential for patient management. GI endoscopists are increasingly involved in measurements and interventions.

Most GI endoscopy suites now include a room largely, if not completely, devoted to the evaluation of GI motility. I was very pleased that Dr. Richard W. McCallum, a leader in this field and our Guest Editor, agreed that it would be a good idea to devote an issue of the *Gastrointestinal Endoscopy Clinics of North America* to gastrointestinal motility. He has assembled a group of expertly authored articles that should be of great interest to endoscopists and clinical gastroenterologists in general. We added two key articles from Dr. Henry P. Parkman's superb September 2007 issue of the *Gastroenterology Clinics of North America* on this topic to round out the current volume. I hope readers will be moved to explore this rapidly developing area, which offers new opportunities for gastrointestinal endoscopists to help more patients who suffer from motility disorders.

Charles J. Lightdale, MD
Department of Medicine
Columbia University Medical Center
161 Fort Washington Avenue, Room 812
New York, NY 10032, USA

E-mail address:
CJL18@columbia.edu (C.J. Lightdale)

Gastrointest Endoscopy Clin N Am 19 (2009) xi
doi:10.1016/j.giec.2009.01.002
1052-5157/09/$ – see front matter
giendo.theclinics.com

Preface

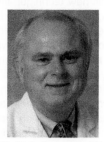

Richard W. McCallum, MD, FACP, FACG
Guest Editor

The goal of this issue of the *Gastrointestinal Endoscopy Clinics of North America* is devoted to gastrointestinal motility and neurogastroenterology to update the busy gastroenterologist/endoscopist on what is new and clinically applicable to their patient care needs and on what can be incorporated into daily clinical challenges. Beginning with the esophagus, Drs. Vaezi and Hong emphasize the importance of not only acid pH monitoring with catheter or Bravo techniques but also the evolving role of esophageal impedance, particularly as a preoperative evaluation when considering Nissen fundoplication measurements. Dr. Fass discusses functional heartburn, which is always challenging and an extremely common aspect of our practice. Finally, a card-carrying esophageal surgeon, Dr. Smith, discusses where we stand today on the indications and results of well-done surgery for gastroesophageal reflux disease.

The next articles address the gastrointestinal (GI) tract by updating topics on the stomach and small bowel. Dr. Parkman emphasizes the evolving role of new methodology for gastric emptying. Although the recent consensus statement by the American Nuclear Medicine Society and the American Neurogastroenterology Motility Society mandated the use of 4-hour gastric emptying as the gold standard, this is not going to happen in clinical community practice and in small towns in this country. As a result, SmartPill technology, which measures transit and pressure in the gut, will become the standard of care in GI practice in the United States and abroad. The article by Drs. Stapleton and Wo shows algorithms for treating the always challenging situation of nausea and vomiting in a patient who sometimes has gastroparesis or, in some cases, functional dyspepsia using an escalating menu with new ways to "reshuffle the deck of cards." In my article with Dr. Hejazi, we address the refractory gastroparetic patient who reaches the upper levels of GI referral, including academic medical centers. There are good options for treatment, although some have been overpromoted, and we need to look at the hard-core data to see what is actually documented and achievable in well-performed studies.

The issue next focuses on constipation and reviews new methodologies for diagnosis, including the role of the previously mentioned SmartPill, and new pharmacology to address the increasing volume of patients wishing to age gracefully. Dr. Sands,

Gastrointest Endoscopy Clin N Am 19 (2009) xiii–xiv
doi:10.1016/j.giec.2009.01.001
giendo.theclinics.com

a surgeon at the Cleveland Clinic in Fort Lauderdale, Florida, brings us exciting news about the role of surgery, particularly sacral nerve stimulation, for fecal incontinence. With regard to advances, this area has been a desert. This new technique involving a sacral nerve stimulator manufactured by the Medtronic Company and being reviewed by the Food and Drug Administration, should be approved within the next year. The surgical approach to constipation not only corrects problems with exit issues of anatomy in the rectum but also could extend to subtotal colectomy and may be helped by the same sacral nerve stimulator initially developed for fecal incontinence. Dr. Rao's article on the treatment and evaluation of colonic and anorectal motility concentrates on slow transit constipation, dyssynergic defecation, and irritable bowel syndrome with constipation. He also presents information on the Rome criteria as a useful guide for making the clinical diagnosis of functional constipation.

The next articles address a large part of any GI practice: functional bowel disorders. Dr. Ringle from Chapel Hill addresses the evolving area of small bowel bacteria overgrowth, which will indeed have a role and will change the paradigm for how we treat functional bowel disorders. Although not being quite the *Helicobacter pylori* of functional bowel disease, small bowel bacteria overgrowth will change the playing field and offer new therapies. Drs. Grover and Drossman offer a comprehensive review of psychopharmacologic and behavioral treatments for functional GI disorders. This review is important because with the evolving understanding in the etiopathogenesis and clinical manifestations of functional GI disorders, the use of centrally acting psychopharmacologic and behavioral treatments is expected to grow.

Finally, the last article, by Drs. Parkman and Orr, presents important information on setting up and running an efficient and practical GI motility laboratory. Proper evaluation of patients who have suspected GI motility disorders is important to ensure a correct diagnosis and to embark on an appropriate plan of treatment. The GI motility laboratory serves as an important area for patient evaluation in gastroenterology and is an essential element in any comprehensive digestive disease program.

In conclusion, this issue of the *Gastrointestinal Endoscopy Clinics of North America* is very timely, authoritative, and an immensely practical asset to your practice. This compilation of articles will bring you up to date with the advances and future directions in GI motility and functional bowel disorders, allowing you to be on the cutting edge for the foreseeable future.

Richard W. McCallum, MD, FACP, FACG
Department of Medicine, Center for GI Nerve & Muscle Function
Division of GI Motility
Kansas University Medical Center
MS 1058, Rainbow Boulevard
Kansas City, KS 66160, USA

E-mail address:
rmccallu@kumc.edu

Gastroesophageal Reflux Monitoring: pH (Catheter and Capsule) and Impedance

Shih-Kuang S. Hong, MD, Michael F. Vaezi, MD, PhD, MSc(Epi)*

KEYWORDS

- GERD • Oropharyngeal devices
- Esophageal impedance monitoring • pH monitoring

Gastroesophageal reflux disease (GERD) is a common disease encountered by primary care physicians and gastroenterologists. Up to 45% of Americans are affected by GERD each month, and the costs related to GERD care can be quite high, reportedly up to $4500 per patient per year.[1] Medications used to treat GERD are some of the most popularly prescribed drugs. Although most patients are initially treated with acid-suppressive therapy, many require diagnostic testing to objectively assess for the presence and degree of esophageal *acid* exposure. Furthermore, the recent increase in prevalence of patients with partial response or lack of response to aggressive acid suppression has raised questions about the role of *less acidic* refluxate in esophageal injury as well as patient symptoms.

Esophageal function testing for GERD has evolved greatly over the last 30 years to allow for greater patient comfort and ambulatory detection of esophageal acid reflux while the patients continue with their normal daily activities. It has progressed from using catheters to evaluate pH to now using a wireless device with sensitivity in the range of 94% to 96% and specificity up to 96% for evaluating GERD.[2] Ambulatory monitoring has also moved beyond detecting acid reflux. Esophageal impedance monitoring, which was developed and studied extensively in recent years, is considered to be the most sensitive ambulatory tool in assessing esophageal refluxate of various composition: acidic, weakly acidic, or nonacidic. The goal of this article is to highlight the utility of pH-metry as well as the role of impedance monitoring in GERD and to discuss the recent advances in ambulatory physiologic monitoring for reflux.

Department of Gastroenterology and Hepatology, Clinical Research, and Center for Swallowing and Esophageal Disorders, Vanderbilt University Medical Center, 1660 TVC, Nashville, TN 37232-5280, USA
* Corresponding author.
E-mail address: michael.vaezi@vanderbilt.edu (M.F. Vaezi).

Gastrointest Endoscopy Clin N Am 19 (2009) 1–22
doi:10.1016/j.giec.2008.12.009
1052-5157/08/$ – see front matter © 2009 Elsevier Inc. All rights reserved.

INDICATIONS FOR pH (± IMPEDANCE) MONITORING

An empiric trial with a proton pump inhibitor (PPI) is the recommended initial approach in all GERD-suspected patients. Response of symptoms to a PPI can be very helpful in establishing the diagnosis of GERD. Various studies have shown that a positive response to an empiric PPI trial (ie, improvement in symptoms) can have a high sensitivity in the diagnosis of GERD but a low and variable specificity.[3] Patients who fail an empiric trial with a PPI should undergo esophageal pH testing to determine whether these symptoms are indeed secondary to GERD (**Box 1**). Patients who do not attain a full response to empiric PPI may also be considered for further esophageal pH testing.

Another group of patients who should undergo esophageal pH testing are those being considered for surgical or endoscopic therapy for reflux (see **Box 1**). In this group of patients, it is essential that abnormal reflux be documented prior to proceeding to an invasive procedure. Additionally, patients who have had surgical or endoscopic reflux therapy but continue to have symptoms postprocedures should also undergo esophageal pH testing to determine if their symptoms are secondary to persistent or recurrent reflux and to help prevent unnecessary therapy with medications such as PPIs or H2 blockers.

Esophageal impedance combined with pH monitoring may be useful in patients with persistent symptoms despite aggressive acid suppression to rule out weakly acidic or nonacidic reflux. This may be especially valuable in patients with atypical symptoms, as it can help correlate times of reflux with the atypical symptoms of cough, chest pain, and wheezing. However, the clinical significance of abnormal non- or weakly acidic reflux in patients on therapy continues to be debated. It is suggested that, in most patients who have tried up to twice a day dosing of PPIs, reflux is most likely not the cause for patients' continued symptoms.[4]

pH MONITORING PARAMETERS

There are six parameters that are often analyzed during esophageal pH monitoring to determine if a patient has abnormal esophageal reflux (**Table 1**) (**Fig. 1**).[5,6] These parameters are often part of every esophageal pH monitoring report, which includes the following:

1. The percent time the pH of the esophagus was less than four over the total monitoring period
2. The percent time the pH was less than four when the patient was supine
3. The percent time the pH was less than four when the patient was upright
4. The total number of reflux episodes
5. The number of reflux episodes greater than 5 minutes
6. The time of the longest reflux episode

Most commonly used parameters assessing for reflux are either percent total time pH < 4[7] or the DeMeester Score (a composite score using the mean values for the above parameters with abnormal being > 22).[8] A study of 53 patients who underwent two 24-hour pH testing periods within 10 days assessed the reproducibility of the above six parameters. The results showed that *total percent time with pH < 4* over the 2 days was the most reproducible parameter. Total percent time with pH < 4 was 85% reproducible compared with 80% reproducibility for percent time pH < 4 while supine, 75% reproducibility for percent time pH < 4 while upright, 69% reproducibility for number of episodes greater than 5 minutes, and 76% reproducibility for longest reflux episode.[7]

> **Box 1**
> **Indications for esophageal pH monitoring**
>
> 1. Patients with typical GERD symptoms who fail 4 weeks of PPI therapy
> 2. Patients with atypical symptoms who fail 6 to 8 weeks of PPI therapy
> 3. Patients being considered for endoscopic or surgical reflux therapy
> 4. Patients who have undergone endoscopic or surgical reflux therapy and who continue to have GERD symptoms

SYMPTOM INDICES

In addition to the actual pH parameters measured during the monitoring period, other indices can correlate patient symptoms to actual reflux observed during pH monitoring. These symptom indices are important components of assessing the relationship between reflux and patients' typical (heartburn, regurgitation) or atypical (chest pain, cough, wheezing) symptoms. The three main symptom indices include the *symptom index (SI), symptom sensitivity index (SSI),* and *symptom association probability (SAP).* They are calculated using the data obtained from 24-hour pH monitoring and using the patient's diary of symptoms. This is why it is important for patients to keep an accurate diary of the timing of their symptoms and to mark their symptoms by pushing the button on the recorder.

The SI is the percentage of symptom episodes that are related to reflux. It is calculated as follows:

(Number of symptom episodes related to pH < 4)/(Total number of symptom episodes) × 100.

The SI is considered positive when it is greater than or equal to 50%. A retrospective study in 1992 examined 153 patients who had undergone 24-hour pH monitoring to determine the value of the SI. The study examined three different groups of patients (patients who had normal 24-hour pH studies and no esophagitis, patients who had abnormal 24-hour pH studies and no esophagitis, and patients with abnormal 24-hour pH studies and esophagitis). They were able to determine that a mean SI for heartburn greater than or equal to 50% had a sensitivity of 93% and specificity of 71% for diagnosing acid reflux.[9] This index is limited by the fact that it does not take into account the total number of reflux episodes that actually occurred.

Another index that does take into account the number of reflux events is SSI. It is calculated as follows:

(Number of symptom episodes related to pH < 4)/(Total number of reflux episodes) × 100.

Table 1 Normal values for 24-h esophageal pH monitoring		
	1974 (Johnson/DeMeester)[5]	1992 (Richter et al)[6]
1. % of Total period pH<4	< 4.2%	< 5.78%
2. % of Supine period pH<4	< 1.2%	< 3.45%
3. % of Upright period pH<4	< 6.3%	< 8.15%
4. Total number of reflux episodes	< 50	< 46
5. Total number of reflux episodes >5 min	≤ 3	< 4
6. Length of longest episode of reflux	< 9.2 min	< 18.45 min

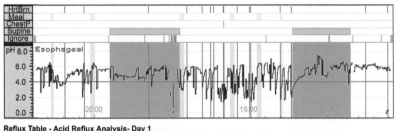

Reflux Table - Acid Reflux Analysis- Day 1

	Total	(Normal)	Upright	(Normal)	Supine	(Normal)
Fraction Time pH <4 ((%))	7.2	5.5	8.9	8.2	4.6	3.0
Number of Refluxes	65		47		18	
Number of Long Refluxes(>5 (min))	5		3		2	
Duration of longest reflux (min)	9		9		9	
Time pH <4 ((min))	95		72		23	

SI Table - Acid Reflux Analysis

	Total
HrtBrn	50.0
Regurg	n/a
ChestP	100.0

Reflux Table - Acid Reflux Analysis- Day 2

	Total	(Normal)	Upright	(Normal)	Supine	(Normal)
Fraction Time pH <4 ((%))	10.9	5.5	14.4	8.2	4.6	3.0
Number of Refluxes	42		37		6	
Number of Long Refluxes(>5 (min))	8		8		1	
Duration of longest reflux (min)	30		20		19	
Time pH <4 ((min))	136		115		20	

SAP Table - Acid Reflux Analysis

	Total
HrtBrn	100.0
Regurg	0.0
ChestP	76.9

Fig. 1. Wireless pH tracing of abnormal esophageal acid exposure. This patient has abnormal upright and supine reflux as the percent time pH < 4 is abnormal. There is a positive symptom index for chest pain and heartburn and positive symptom association probability for heartburn.

This index is considered positive when it is greater than or equal to 10%. There is a high degree of correlation between the SI and SSI,[10] but the discordance rate could be as high as 33% (ie, a high SI and low SSI or low SI and high SSI).

The most recent and scientific index is the SAP. It is calculated by dividing the total 24-hour pH recording data into 2-minute segments. In each 2-minute segment, it is determined if there are reflux events and if there are reported symptoms. These data are then summarized into a 2 × 2 table. The four fields in the table are as follows:

Positive symptom Positive reflux	Positive symptom Negative reflux
Negative symptom Positive reflux	Negative symptom Negative reflux

The association between reflux and symptoms is then calculated using Fisher's exact test. An SAP greater than 95% is considered positive and indicates that the probability of the association of reflux and symptoms occurring by chance is less than 5%. A high SAP suggests that a patient's symptoms are likely secondary to reflux. A study examining 184 pH-monitoring tracings found that the SAP showed an 11% discordance rate with the SI and a 15% discordance rate with the SSI.[11]

One study attempted to compare the three indices by calculating their sensitivities and specificities. Taghavi and colleagues performed 24-hour pH monitoring in 28 patients with heartburn and then measured their response to omeprazole with

a questionnaire.[12] Using this method, they determined the sensitivities and specificities as follows:

	Sensitivity	Specificity
SAP	65.22%	73.33%
SSI	73.91%	73.33%
SI	34.78%	80%

The findings from this study suggest that these indices fall short of being the "gold
standard," and further refinement is still needed. The same indices may be used in
impedance monitoring to assess the relationship between non- or weakly acidic reflux
events and patients' symptoms. In this case, the analysis would be the same except
that the comparator would not be for events with pH < 4 but for events occurring
between pH 4 and 7 for weakly acidic events and above pH 7 for nonacidic events.
It is important to note that these indices continue to be useful in linking symptoms
and actual reflux; however, their role in predicting response to therapy is uncertain.

TYPES OF ELECTRODES

Currently, there are two main types of pH-monitoring devices in common clinical use:
the traditional catheter-based monitor (**Fig. 2**) and the wireless pH monitor (**Fig. 3**).
Most recently an oropharyngeal pH catheter (Restech) has also become available
(**Fig. 4**). Although clinical experience with this device is limited, it shows promise
and ongoing studies may position it in a better light in the future. Impedance monitoring uses a catheter device, similar to that used in traditional catheter-based pH
monitoring, positioned transnasally.

PATIENT PREPARATION

Preparation for the pH- and impedance-monitoring devices is similar. The procedures
are performed in the fasting state. If the test is to be performed off therapy, patients
should be instructed to stop their acid-suppressive medications before testing. It is
recommended that PPIs be stopped at least 7 days before the study. H2 blockers
should be stopped 3 days before the study. Antacids should be stopped at least

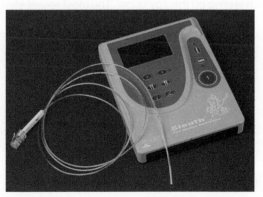

Fig. 2. Catheter-based pH monitoring system. Recorder and catheter are shown. (*Courtesy of*
Anne Rayner, Nashville, TN.)

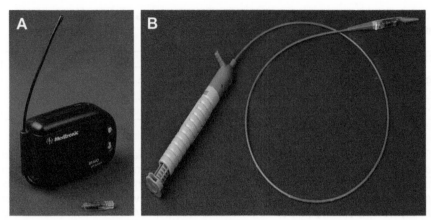

Fig. 3. (A) Wireless pH capsule and recording device. (B) Wireless pH capsule introducing device. (*Courtesy of* Anne Rayner, Nashville, TN.)

6 to 12 hours before the study. If studies are to be performed on therapy, patients should be instructed to continue with their acid-suppressive therapy up to and including the day of testing. Wireless pH capsules are often placed endoscopically, but these capsules usually monitor esophageal pH for 48 hours rather than 24 hours as a standard pH catheter would. It should be noted that wireless pH monitors can be placed without using endoscopy or sedation.

The decision on whether to perform pH or impedance monitoring *off* or *on* acid-suppressive therapy is controversial. One study retrospectively examined 250 patients who had undergone pH testing while on PPI therapy. This study found that most of the patients had normal pH monitoring data, showing that the clinical yield for pH monitoring while *on* PPI therapy is low.[4] Another study examined patients while *off* and *on* PPI therapy over an extended monitoring time of 96 hours using wireless pH monitoring.[13] The study examined 18 patients with atypical symptoms off therapy for 24 hours and then on twice-a-day PPI therapy for another 72 hours. They found that most of the patients (six out of seven) who had an abnormal pH in the first 24 hours did have normalization of the esophageal pH over the next 72 hours. This study showed that it is feasible to perform extended periods of pH testing while off and on therapy if using the wireless device; however, similar to the above study, they confirmed that the clinical yield for such testing on therapy is low. The most recent study suggests that if

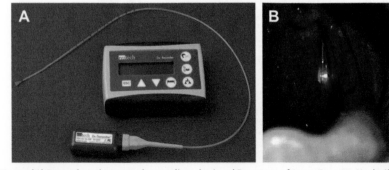

Fig. 4. (A) Restech catheter and recording device. (*Courtesy of* Anne Rayner, Nashville, TN.) (B) Oropharyngeal pH probe with transmitter and LED tip in the posterior aspect of the mouth.

only one test is to be performed, then impedance monitoring on therapy results in more clinically valuable information than does pH monitoring off therapy.[14]

CATHETER-BASED pH MONITORING

Antimony catheters are the most commonly used pH catheters in clinical practice. In the past glass catheters were used, but they went out of favor because they were less comfortable and more expensive. Glass catheters may be more suitable for basic science research, because they tend to react more quickly to pH changes, provide a more linear response, and have less recording drift than do antimony electrodes. Both types of electrode have shown similar results when used clinically.

Positioning the pH Catheter

Distal esophagus

The pH probe is typically placed about 5 cm above the lower esophageal sphincter (LES), because this is felt to be the ideal location that will prevent the probe from being displaced into the stomach during swallowing. One study looked at the importance of placing the probe 5 cm above the LES.[15] The authors used a single catheter with two sensors that were positioned such that one sensor was 5 cm above the LES and one sensor was 10 cm above the LES. The results showed significant differences in all six parameters of the Johnson and DeMeester score in patients who had pathologic reflux. The sensor at 10 cm detected less acid reflux than didthe sensor at 5 cm. Distal esophageal pH monitoring data suggest that there is a stepwise increase in the degree of esophageal acid exposure across the "spectrum" of GERD.[16]

Alternate sites

Proximal esophageal probes are similarly positioned at either 10 cm or 15 cm above this manometric location. Hypopharyngeal pH catheter placement is more commonly used in research and is typically based on the location of the upper esophageal sphincter (UES) determined manometrically. The hypopharyngeal pH catheter is typically positioned at 1 cm or 2 cm above UES. However, pH probes in this area are prone to drying and causing an artificial drop in the detected pH (ie, pseudo-reflux). Clinical studies using proximal and hypopharyngeal pH catheters are usually conducted in patients with atypical manifestations of GERD, such as asthma, laryngitis, chest pain, or cough.[17] For example, Jacob and colleagues[18] demonstrated increased proximal esophageal acid exposure in a subset of patients with laryngitis suspected to be GERD-related. Koufman and colleagues[19] found that seven of the 16 patients (44%) with laryngeal symptoms had abnormal hypopharyngeal reflux events predominantly in the upright position. Similarly, later studies by Shaker and colleagues[20] and Ylitalo and colleagues[21] using hypopharyngeal pH probes showed increased prevalence of pharyngeal reflux in patients with posterior laryngitis compared with that in control subjects and GERD patients. Additionally, Oelschlager and colleagues[22] evaluated 76 patients with respiratory symptoms suspected to be GERD-related. Their findings suggest that GERD may be the likely cause of patients' atypical symptoms when both pH monitoring and laryngoscopy are abnormal.

While pretherapy prevalence studies suggest that abnormal reflux events may be present in up to 53% of patients with reflux laryngitis,[17] they do not establish causal relationship. This may be due to poor sensitivity of pH monitoring. Vaezi and colleagues[23] tested reproducibility and reliability of the proximal and distal esophageal pH probe in 32 patients (11 controls, 10 with distal reflux and 11 with both proximal and distal reflux). They found that the sensitivity of distal and proximal pH probes were 70% and 55%, respectively. Additionally, a 2003 study by Shaker and colleagues[24] showed the number and duration of hypopharyngeal reflux events to be similar between the control subjects and patients with reflux laryngitis and vasomotor rhinitis. Some reflux into the hypopharynx may be a normal phenomenon. In a 2003 study by Bilgen and colleagues,[25] there was no significant difference in hypopharyngeal acid exposure between 23 healthy individuals and 36 patients with laryngeal signs and symptoms. Additionally, Maldonado and colleagues[26] found a 10% prevalence of abnormal hypopharyngeal pH in normal subjects. Given this uncertainty, it is important to standardize esophageal reflux parameters in the hypopharynx to better understand the causal relationship between reflux and laryngeal disease.

The most recent catheter-based pH probe is one that places the catheter tip in the oropharynx (Restech Dx-pH) (see **Fig. 4**). The Dx-pH Measurement System is a new, potentially more sensitive, and minimally invasive device for detection of acid reflux in the posterior oropharynx. It uses a nasopharyngeal catheter able to measure pH in either liquid or aerosolized droplets. The probe is a 1.5-mm-diameter oropharyngeal catheter with a wireless digital ZigBee transmitter on the shirt collar. The catheter employs a 3.2-mm teardrop tip to aid in insertion and to ensure that the sensor is positioned in the airway (see **Fig. 4**A). The tip has a colored light emitting diode (LED) for oral visualization (see **Fig. 4**B). The special circuitry of this device prevents the inclusion of dry-out related "pseudo-reflux" events in the data. Comparative catheter responsiveness as well as clinical studies with this device are currently ongoing.

Advantages/Disadvantages of Catheter-Based pH Testing

One advantage of the catheter-based pH monitoring systems is that they have a higher sampling rate compared with that of wireless systems (this is especially the case with the new Restech pH device), thus giving them the ability to more accurately detect shorter reflux episodes. The traditional catheter-based systems have a sampling rate of 4 to 5 seconds, wireless based systems have a sampling rate of 6 seconds, and Restech catheters have a sampling rate of 0.5 seconds. The ideal sampling rate to detect the highest number of reflux episodes is 1 Hz, which is higher than that of both the traditional catheter-based systems (0.2–0.25 Hz) and wireless systems (0.17 Hz) but similar to that of the Restech system (2 Hz). One of the major disadvantages of catheter-based pH monitoring is that it may prevent patients from performing their typical daily activities. One study prospectively compared 50 patients with catheter-based pH monitoring and wireless pH monitoring.[27] The patients with the wireless probe reported significantly less problems with interference in their daily activities, sleep, and eating. Patients with the wireless monitor did report significantly more chest discomfort. One other possible disadvantage of catheter-based testing is that it can only be done for 24 hours, whereas wireless pH testing is routinely performed for 48 hours.

WIRELESS pH MONITORING

The wireless pH monitor currently in use is the Bravo capsule (Medtronic, Minneapolis, MN) (see **Fig. 3**). The Bravo capsule contains an antimony pH electrode with an internal reference electrode, a battery, and a transmitter all encapsulated in epoxy. It measures 6 mm × 5.5 mm × 25 mm. The data from the capsule are transmitted at a frequency of 433 MHz and the capsule measures pH at 6-second sampling intervals. The two main advantages of this device are (1) no catheters in the patient's throat or nose, thus reducing discomfort and improving adherence to daily activity; (2) longer monitoring (usually 48 hours and up to 96 hours), thus taking into account the day-to-day variability of reflux in a given patient. Because of these advantages, this mode of esophageal pH monitoring is considered to be superior to catheter monitoring due to improved sensitivity and clinical yield.

Positioning the Capsule in the Esophagus

Unlike the pH catheter, which is placed 5 cm above the manometric LES, the wireless capsule is placed 6 cm above the squamocolumnar junction (SCJ). Once attached to the esophageal mucosa, the pH capsule is not subject to migration or displacement into the stomach with swallowing as with the pH catheter. The distance of 6 cm was chosen based on a study that examined the distance of the SCJ from the high-pressure zone of the LES.[28] This study compared the distance of the SCJ from the high-pressure zone using manometry to identify the high-pressure zone and endoscopy to identify and clip the SCJ. Fluoroscopy was then used to compare the distance in normal patients and distance in patients with a hiatal hernia. The average distance between the SCJ and the LES high-pressure zone was found to be approximately 1.1 cm. Thus, the pH catheter is usually placed about 5 cm above LES and the wireless capsule is placed about 6 cm above the SCJ (which is on average 1.1 cm distal to the LES). As the wireless capsule is placed in relation to the SCJ, this can sometimes be difficult to establish in patients with Barrett esophagus. In this group of patients, pH monitoring is seldom required, since, by definition, these patients have reflux disease; however, if these patients need pH testing, conventional catheter-based pH testing may be reasonable to avoid inappropriate placement of the pH capsule. Wireless capsules can be used in these patients, but other methods would have to be employed for placement. There are three ways this can be done: (1) Placing the capsule transnasally using manometry to identify the LES (higher discomfort to patients and technically more difficult); (2) Orally determining the LES location using manometry and then placing the wireless capsule orally; or (3) Identifying the SCJ based on the area of penetration of submucosal vessels in the distal esophagus (preferred).

After the capsule is placed, patients should be instructed to keep a diary of times for meals and snacks, times for when the patient is in a supine position, and times for reflux symptoms. Patients can also push a button on the recorder to mark symptoms. The diary information can later be inserted into the capsule recording when it is being reviewed to help correlate with times of reflux.

Some patients may complain of chest pain. If the chest pain is severe, a chest x-ray should be performed to rule out an esophageal perforation. If there is no evidence of a perforation, then the pain can be treated conservatively using viscous lidocaine or sucralfate (Carafate). In 2% to 5% of patients, pain may be severe enough to necessitate capsule removal endoscopically. Typically, capsules fall off by themselves after 5 days. If the capsule needs to be removed endoscopically, this can be accomplished using a polypectomy snare. The polypectomy snare should be placed loosely around the capsule and should be pushed back and forth against the capsule. If this does not dislodge the capsule, then the capsule can be dislodged by tightening the snare at the base of the capsule. The snare should be as close to the capsule as possible. The endoscope should not be used to push the capsule off the esophageal wall, because this can cause stripping of the mucosa.

Data Interpretation

Data are interpreted similarly to the data from a pH catheter. The same parameters that are used for the Johnson and DeMeester score are used. The main difference is that the normal percent total exposure time to pH < 4 is less than 5.3% instead of the 4.2% used in pH catheter-based studies. This value was determined by a study that compared wireless pH studies in 44 healthy patients and 41 patients with

GERD over an extended monitoring period (36–48 h). In normal patients, the 95th percentile for time the pH < 4 over 36 to 48 hours was 5.3%.[29]

One of the other advantages of the wireless pH capsule is its ability to record pH for a longer period of time: 48 hours (or longer) versus 24 hours. One study found that the symptom association probability increased by 15% when using 48-hour pH testing.[30] Furthermore, given day-to-day variability in esophageal acid exposure,[29] a longer monitoring period may increase the sensitivity of wireless pH monitoring. Prolonged pH testing up to 96 hours can also be performed using the wireless pH monitoring system. This can allow for testing while off and on therapy to see if acid-suppressive therapy is effective.

There are some disadvantages to wireless pH monitoring. One of the disadvantages is early capsule detachment. It was initially reported that this could happen in up to 12% of capsules that were attached. This has improved since the manufacturer made some improvements to the capsule delivery device. Early capsule detachment can result in false-positive pH parameters due to exposure of the capsule to gastric acidity. The typical pattern to recognize for this condition is one of a sharp and prolonged pH change to near pH 1 with subsequent recovery in minutes or hours to pH greater than seven (**Fig. 5**).

MULTICHANNEL INTRALUMINAL IMPEDANCE

Until recently, testing for GERD was largely based on 24-hour ambulatory pH monitoring.[31] When patients are on PPIs, reflux events are often "non- or weakly" acidic and, therefore, undetectable by conventional pH monitoring.[32] The ability of multichannel intraluminal impedance (MII) as a technique to evaluate esophageal function promises to further enhance the detection of esophageal abnormalities.

MII uses inherent conductive or resistive properties of the intraluminal bolus (liquid, gas, or mixed) to examine the presence and transit of the bolus in the esophageal lumen. Two variations of MII have been introduced for clinical use: combined MII and pH monitoring (MII-pH) and combined MII and esophageal manometry. We specifically focus on the role of impedance in combination with pH-metry in evaluation of refractory GERD and discuss the principles of impedance testing, the clinical utilities, and the limitations of this device.

Basic Principles

Impedance is a measure of total resistance to the alternating current flow. In MII testing, impedance is measured between two electrodes spaced 2 cm apart (ie,

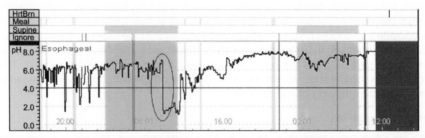

Fig. 5. This pH tracing shows a wireless pH capsule that has dislodged from the esophagus and fallen into the stomach. The sharp drop in the pH (area within the oval) represents the capsule falling into the stomach. The pH then rises back up, representing the passage of the capsule into the small bowel. If not identified and omitted from the analysis, this would result in a false-positive pH reading and patient misclassification.

impedance-measuring segment). The electrodes are connected to an impedance voltage transducer outside the body via thin wires that run the length of the catheter. The voltage generated by the transducer is limited to produce at most 8 µA of current, which is 1000-fold below the threshold for cardiac stimulation.[33] The actual current generated is dependent on the electrical conductive or resistive properties of the material in contact with the two electrodes completing the electrical circuit. Impedance, expressed in ohms, is the ratio of voltage to the current. The impedance tracing produced by MII testing represents the average of all impedance values in the cross-sectional area of the esophagus between the two electrodes.

Impedance is inversely related to the cross-sectional area of the esophagus and the electrical conductivity of the intraluminal substance being measured.[33] Electrical conductivity is dependent on the ionic concentration of the surrounding material. Therefore, substances with high ionic concentration, such as liquid swallows or gastroesophageal reflux (GER), have high conductance and low impedance. Conversely, substances with low ionic concentration, such as air or gas refluxate, have low conductance and high impedance. Mixed (liquid and gas) bolus exhibits characteristics of both.[34,35] Thus, with impedance, esophageal intraluminal contents can be differentiated as liquid, gas, or mixed bolus.[34,35]

Characteristic esophageal impedance tracing correlating with a liquid bolus movement across the impedance-measuring segment was validated with simultaneous videofluoroscopy (**Fig. 6**).[36,37] At baseline, the esophagus is a narrow, empty tube, and the baseline impedance is determined by the esophageal mucosa in contact with the impedance-measuring segment. As the liquid bolus reaches the impedance-measuring segment, the esophagus expands and impedance rises sharply because of the air in front of the bolus head. This is followed by a rapid drop in impedance as liquid bolus passes the measuring segment (see **Fig. 6**). Bolus entry is considered to be at 50% impedance drop from baseline to nadir, and bolus exit is considered to be a 50% rise from nadir to baseline.[38] The impedance stays at nadir as long as the bolus is present on the impedance-measuring segment. Bolus is cleared with esophageal contraction and lumen narrowing. This results in transient impedance elevation ("overshoot") above the baseline before stabilizing.

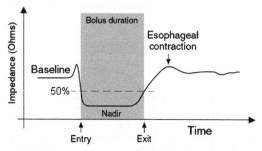

Fig. 6. Characteristic impedance tracing of a liquid bolus. At baseline, the esophagus is a narrow, empty tube, and the impedance is determined by the electrical properties of the esophageal mucosa. As the bolus reaches the impedance-measuring segment, the esophagus expands, and the impedance rises sharply due to the air in front of the bolus head. This is followed by a rapid drop in impedance, as higher conductive liquid bolus passes the measuring segment. Bolus entry is considered to be at the 50% drop in impedance from baseline and bolus exit at the 50% rise from the nadir. The impedance stays at nadir as long as the bolus is present on the impedance-measuring segment. Esophageal contraction causes lumen narrowing and passage of bolus, resulting in transient impedance elevation ("overshoot") above the baseline before returning to baseline.

A typical MII catheter consists of multiple impedance-measuring segments (ie, multichannel) mounted 5 cm apart on a 2.1-mm-diameter polyvinyl catheter (Sandhill Scientific, Inc, Denver, CO). Multichannel impedance allows assessment of esophageal bolus transit. The direction of bolus movement is determined based on the time sequence of bolus entry and exit through different impedance-measuring segments. For example, antegrade bolus movement (ie, swallow) is shown by bolus entry progressing from proximal to distal impedance-measuring segments over time (**Fig. 7**). However, retrograde bolus movement (ie, reflux) is shown (**Fig. 8**) by bolus entry progressing from distal to proximal impedance-measuring segments followed by proximal to distal bolus exit (ie, clearance) over time.[38] The ability of MII to accurately assess bolus transit has been validated with simultaneous videofluoroscopy.[39]

COMBINED MII-pH

Impedance testing is usually performed in combination with pH monitoring. Combined, they provide complementary information and afford better assessment of GERD. MII-pH allows detection of GER of various consistencies—both acid and nonacid as well as liquid and nonliquid events.[38] The role of nonacid reflux in GERD has gained recognition in the past decade.[40–42] It is shown that while up to 90% of patients with erosive esophagitis will achieve endoscopic healing, 35% will have persistent symptoms despite PPI therapy.[43] In a study of patients with persistent symptoms refractory to acid suppression, Shay and colleagues found that in some patients the refractory symptoms may be due to nonacid reflux.[44] Other nonacid reflux monitoring devices have limitations and therefore are not widely used. For example, scintigraphic methods are costly, require radiation exposure, and are insensitive because they monitor only a short time period.[45] Similarly, Bilitec 2000 (bilirubin monitoring device) measures only bile refluxate and may miss more than 90% of nonacid reflux that is nonbilious.[33,46]

The combined MII-pH catheter is a thin flexible 2.1-mm polyvinyl catheter (Sandhill Scientific, Inc) similar to the standard pH catheter. On this catheter are six impedance-measuring segments (four distal and two proximal) and a pH sensor (**Fig. 9**). It is placed into the esophagus transnasally and positioned so that the pH sensor is 5 cm above the LES. The impedance-measuring segments are located on the catheter

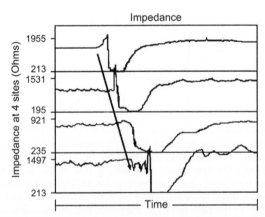

Fig. 7. Multichannel impedance measurement of antegrade (swallow) liquid bolus movement. The antegrade direction of the bolus movement (swallow) is shown by bolus entry progression from proximal to distal impedance-measuring segments over time (*arrow*).

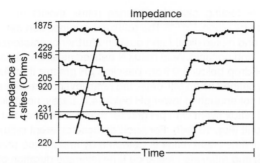

Fig. 8. Multichannel impedance measurement of retrograde (reflux) liquid bolus movement. The retrograde direction of the bolus movement (reflux) is shown by bolus entry progression from distal to proximal impedance-measuring segments over time (*arrow*) followed by proximal to distal bolus exit progression over time (or clearance).

such that, when properly placed in the esophagus, impedance at 3, 5, 7, 9, 15, and 17 cm above the LES is measured.

The MII-pH test is performed in a similar manner to 24-hour ambulatory pH monitoring. The patient is instructed to fast 4 to 6 hours before the MII-pH probe is placed. During the monitoring period, the patient is instructed to perform normal daily activities, consume his or her usual diet, and keep a diary of symptoms, meal times, time of lying down for sleep, time of rising in the morning, and time of acid-suppression medication. The patient returns the following day to have the probe removed and diary reviewed. The MII-pH data are downloaded and analyzed using a software program.

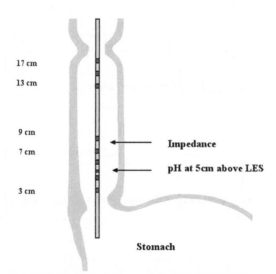

Fig. 9. MII-pH. A combined MII-pH catheter is a thin, flexible, 2.1-mm polyvinyl catheter (Sandhill Scientific, Inc, Denver, CO) similar to a standard pH catheter. On this catheter are 6 impedance-measuring segments (4 distal and 2 proximal) and a pH sensor. It is placed into the esophagus transnasally and positioned so that the pH sensor is 5 cm above LES. The impedance-measuring segments are located on the catheter such that when properly placed in the esophagus, impedance at 3, 5, 7, 9, 15, and 17 cm above LES are measured. (LES, lower esophageal sphincter.)

Combined MII/pH testing can characterize reflux events in various ways not possible with pH-metry alone.[38,39,46] The refluxate composition can be differentiated among liquid, gas, and mixed (liquid and gas) and further characterized as acid, weak acid, acid re-reflux, and nonacid. Acid reflux is defined as an MII-detected reflux event with associated pH drop below 4.0 from baseline pH greater than 4.0 (**Fig. 10**, right). Weak acid reflux is defined as an MII-detected reflux event that causes more than one unit of pH drop but not enough to lower pH below 4.0. Lastly, nonacid reflux is defined as an MII-detected reflux event with pH greater than 4.0 that does not cause pH drop by more than one unit (**Fig. 10**, left). For each of these different reflux types, refluxate presence time (total time liquid reflux is detected by impedance-measuring segment at 5 cm above LES) and refluxate clearance time (average duration of liquid reflux detected by impedance-measuring segment at 5 cm above LES) are also calculated. In addition, proximal extent is determined as the most proximal measuring segment reached by the liquid refluxate.

Combined MII/pH results are interpreted based on the normal values established by Shay and colleagues[47] in a multicenter study of 60 healthy volunteers without reflux symptoms. Based on the 95th percentile as the upper limit of normal, they proposed

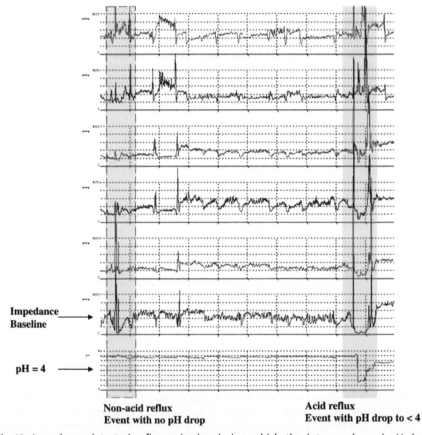

Impedance Baseline

pH = 4

Non-acid reflux
Event with no pH drop

Acid reflux
Event with pH drop to < 4

Fig. 10. Impedance-detected reflux episodes during which the intraesophageal pH drops from greater than 4 to less than 4 are considered acid (*right*), whereas impedance-detected reflux episodes during which the intraesophageal pH remains greater than 4.0 are considered non-acid (*left*).

normal total distal reflux to be total reflux events less than or equal to 73, acid reflux events less than or equal to 55, weak acid reflux events less than or equal to 26, and nonacid reflux events less than or equal to one. Similarly, normal total proximal reflux events were defined as total reflux events less than or equal to 31, acid reflux events less than or equal to 28, weak acid reflux events less than or equal to one, and nonacid reflux events less than or equal to one (**Table 2**). These normative data were established *off* acid-suppression therapy. Because MII-pH is most likely to be used for symptomatic patients on acid-suppression therapy, on-therapy normal values are needed. Studying the effects of omeprazole on 2-hour postprandial GER, Vela and colleagues found that PPI therapy reduced acid reflux episodes with proportional increase in nonacid reflux, the net result of which was an unchanged total number of reflux episodes on or off therapy.[32] In another study, Jeske and colleagues studied preoperative administration of esomeprazole in 21 healthy volunteers and found that while pH of gastric contents was significantly higher and gastric content volume was significantly lower with PPI administration compared with those of placebo, no significant difference was found with respect to number of acid or total reflux episodes per person, duration of reflux, or barrier pressure.[48] However, Tutuian and colleagues showed that PPI therapy does reduce the total number of reflux events, suggesting that the upper limit of normal for patients on twice daily PPI therapy should be 48 reflux events.[49]

In 2006, some investigators used SAP and SI for reflux-symptom correlation in patients undergoing MII-pH.[50] In a 2006 study evaluating the additional yield of impedance over pH-metry in 60 patients off therapy, Bredenoord and colleagues[51] found that positive SAP increased from 66.7% to 77.1% (*P*<.05) by adding MII to pH monitoring. Thus, MII by detecting SAP in nonacid reflux and weakly acid reflux helps to increase the yield in patients with symptoms attributable to reflux.

CLINICAL APPLICATIONS OF MII-pH

MII-pH is studied in the *pediatric population* to evaluate the role of acid and nonacid reflux in those with chronic respiratory symptoms, such as recurrent apnea, aspiration pneumonia, and asthma.[52–55] GERD is associated with respiratory symptoms in children,[56] and in refractory cases nonacid reflux has been implicated.[53] In one of the first studies using MII-pH, Skopnik and colleagues[54] noted a significant number of nonacid reflux episodes in 17 infants with respiratory symptoms that were not detected by pH monitoring alone. In a 2004 study of MII-pH in 28 children with persistent respiratory symptoms on PPI therapy, nonacid reflux represented 45% of all reflux episodes; multivariate analysis demonstrated a stronger association between respiratory symptoms and nonacid reflux than that with acid reflux events.[53] A strong relationship between acid and nonacid GER and respiratory abnormalities was also demonstrated

Table 2
Normal values for combined MII-pH (95th percentile)[47]

	Distal Reflux Events					Proximal Reflux Events				
	Total	Acid	Weak acid	Nonacid	Acid re-reflux	Total	Acid	Weak acid	Nonacid	Acid re-reflux
Total	73	55	26	1	4	31	28	12	1	2
Upright	67	52	24	1	4	29	25	11	1	2
Recumbent	7	5	4	0	1	3	2	1	0	0

in a study reported by Wenzl and colleagues.[57] In a group of 22 children who presented with repetitive regurgitation and chronic respiratory symptoms, impedance recorded 364 episodes of reflux, of which only 11.4% were acidic. Of these reflux events, 312 (85%; 12% of which were acidic) could be associated with irregular breathing. Analysis of the polysomnographic recording revealed 165 episodes of apnea, of which 30% were associated with a reflux episode. The majority (78%) of reflux episodes were detected by impedance only.[57]

In adults, MII-pH has been used for evaluation of typical and atypical GER symptoms refractory to aggressive acid-suppression therapy.[58–60] In a European study from 2007, Bajbouj and colleagues[61] examined the diagnostic yield of MII-pH in patients with atypical GER symptoms. Forty-one patients with atypical GERD symptoms were included in their study and were examined by endoscopy, dual-channel pH-metry, and impedance monitoring; all patients were asked to hold PPI therapy for 2 weeks. A total of 26 patients (63.4%) had pathologic findings in any method. The highest diagnostic yield was achieved by combined 24-hour MII-pH (61.0%), followed by solely impedance measurement (48.8%), distal pH-metry (29.3%), endoscopy (22.8%), and proximal pH-metry (17.1%).

In refractory GERD patients on PPI therapy, MII-pH findings suggest a possible, but not fully established, role for nonacid reflux.[32,62] Vela and colleagues[32] performed MII-pH on 12 GERD patients before and after 7 days of omeprazole therapy. They found a significant decrease in acid reflux from 45% before therapy to 3% after therapy ($P = .02$). However, this was offset by an increase in nonacid reflux events (from 55% to 97%, $P = .03$), and as a result the total number of reflux episodes remained the same. Interestingly, they found that heartburn and acid taste were also produced by nonacid reflux events. Similar findings were reported by Tamhankar and colleagues,[62] who found that 7 days of twice-daily omeprazole therapy did not reduce the total number of reflux episodes. In this study, acid reflux episodes decreased from 63% to 2.1% ($P<.0001$), but nonacid reflux episodes increased from 15% to 76% ($P<.0001$). These studies suggest, as expected, that PPI therapy converts acid reflux to less-acid or nonacid reflux. As a result, although PPI therapy reduces acid reflux events, the total number of reflux events is unchanged. The potential implication of this finding is that nonacid reflux may still play an important role in persistent reflux symptoms that are refractory to PPI therapy.

Several studies have aimed at identifying determinants of reflux perception in patients on PPI therapy by means of ambulatory MII-pH monitoring.[63–65] Tutuian and colleagues[64] studied 120 patients with persistent symptoms on acid-suppressive therapy; 3547 reflux episodes (84.3% nonacid, 50.6% mixed composition) were recorded, of which 468 (13.2%) were symptomatic. Based on multivariable analysis, they found that reflux episodes extending proximally and having a mixed (liquid-gas) composition are significantly associated with symptoms, irrespective of whether the pH is acidic or nonacidic. Zerbib and colleagues[65] studied 20 patients on double-dosed PPIs and found that most of the reflux events were asymptomatic (75.5%). They found with their analysis that the only factor associated with reflux perception was the high proximal extent of the refluxate. Compared with regurgitation, reflux episodes associated with heartburn were more frequently pure liquid and acidic, had a lower nadir pH, were more frequently preceded by acid reflux episodes, and had a longer reflux bolus clearance time.[65] Emerenziani and colleagues[63] in their evaluation of 32 nonerosive reflux disease (NERD) patients and 20 esophagitis patients found that in NERD patients, the presence of gas in the refluxate significantly increased the probability of reflux perception. These patients were also more sensitive to less acidic reflux than esophagitis patients.

One prospective study recently assessed the surgical outcome of symptomatic patients despite PPI therapy who had a positive SI with nonacid reflux by impedance.[66] This study reported that, after a mean follow-up of 14 months, 94% of patients reported resolution or improvement of their symptoms. However, this important finding requires confirmation by controlled randomized trials, which are ongoing.

The subgroup of patients presenting with "GERD-related laryngitis" is a special challenge. These patients present with such symptoms as hoarseness, globus, and sore throat and are usually diagnosed based on findings of an ear, nose, and throat specialist on laryngoscopic examination. However, poor specificity of laryngoscopic findings coupled with poor and unpredictable symptom response (60%–98%) to aggressive PPI therapy makes these cases a diagnostic dilemma.[67] One published study evaluated the role of MII-pH in patients with reflux laryngitis.[41] Kawamura and colleagues[41] performed esophageal and pharyngeal MII-pH on 10 patients with reflux laryngitis, 11 patients with GERD, and 10 healthy control subjects. They found that the overall number of pharyngeal reflux events was less than half of that in the proximal esophagus and mostly consisted of gas. All three groups had similar pharyngeal nonacid gas reflux, but the reflux laryngitis group had a significantly higher frequency of weakly acidic gas reflux, defined as a pH drop greater than one but not below 4.0. This pH drop might have been due to a small-volume liquid acid reflux that was masked by the gas.[41] This study suggests that, in patients with reflux laryngitis, hypopharyngeal reflux of gaseous acid may be important. However, this finding was not confirmed by a 2005 study at our institution. We completed a cohort study of 21 patients with suspected GERD-related laryngeal symptoms refractory to twice-daily PPIs.[68] All patients underwent ambulatory 24-hour MII-pH testing: 12 patients were tested on therapy, and nine were off therapy. The results showed that the total number of (acid and nonacid) distal esophageal reflux events was well within normal limits for all patients.[68] Additionally, no hypopharyngeal reflux events (acid or nonacid) were found in any of the cohort. As expected, distal esophageal acid reflux was more prevalent in the off-therapy group, whereas nonacid reflux was more common in the on-therapy group. Our data suggest that the cause of "suspected reflux laryngitis" in this group is unlikely to be related to acid or nonacid reflux events. The relative insignificance of reflux in causing persistent laryngeal symptoms after a 4-month double-dose PPI therapy was further confirmed in a surgical study in which patients were offered surgical fundoplication or continued PPI usage.[69] After 12 months, only 10% (1/10) of patients in the surgical group and 7% (1/15) of patients in the medical group had improvement in laryngeal symptoms. Thus, the argument for any type of reflux as the cause of refractory laryngeal symptoms appears tenuous but is a point of contention with continued investigation.

In 2006, 2 large, multicenter studies reported their findings of MII-pH in patients on and off therapy with PPIs.[50,70] In a European study,[50] 150 patients were included; of those, 79 were off therapy and 71 were on therapy and the reflux-symptom correlation was assessed by SAP. In patients off therapy, the authors found that positive SAP was present in 55% of symptomatic patients (41/74; 5 patients did not have symptoms), including 31% with acid reflux, 4% with nonacid reflux, and 20% with both acid and nonacid reflux. On the other hand, in patients on therapy, positive SAP was found in 37% of symptomatic patients (22/60; 11 patients did not have symptoms), including 5% with acid reflux, 17% with nonacid reflux, and 15% with both acid and nonacid reflux. Furthermore, the investigators also found that the most common symptoms associated with nonacid reflux were regurgitation and cough. The implications of this study are that even though SAP is reduced by PPIs (55% versus 37%), reflux continues to occur to patients on therapy and that most of such reflux episodes are nonacid and associated with symptoms.

In a different study,[70] 168 patients with persistent symptoms on therapy were evaluated by MII-pH using SI to assess reflux-symptom correlation. Of them, 144 (86%) patients recorded symptoms and positive SI was present in 48%; 11% had acid reflux, and 37% had nonacid reflux. Furthermore, the authors assessed the relative importance of acid and nonacid reflux in typical and atypical symptoms. They found that of 171 typical GERD symptoms, positive SI was present with acid reflux in 11% and nonacid reflux in 31%, whereas 58% of symptoms had negative SI. On the other hand, of 131 atypical symptoms, positive SI was present with acid reflux in 3% and nonacid reflux in 19%, whereas 78% of symptoms had negative SI. This study demonstrated that in patients with refractory symptoms on PPI therapy, some (31% typical and 19% atypical) may have reflux events of nonacid reflux associated with continued symptoms; however, the majority (58% typical and 78% atypical) of symptoms on therapy have no correlation with reflux of any kind, acid, nonacid, liquid, or gas.

LIMITATIONS

MII-pH is a useful tool in diagnosing GERD, but impedance testing has some imperfections related to pathologic changes in the esophageal mucosa, such as Barrett esophagus or esophagitis.[71] These changes may cause the baseline impedance values to be very low and detection of the bolus movement in the esophagus to be difficult. In addition, changes in the esophageal mucosa may also impair the esophageal motility and esophageal transit, leading to fluid retention in the esophagus. Domingues and colleagues[72] have demonstrated significantly lower postprandial impedance values among GERD patients with mild esophagitis than those among healthy controls, indicating the presence of liquid residues in the esophagus. Another study observed that patients with esophageal dysmotility had low baseline impedance values in the distal esophagus, which were likely caused by fluid retention within the esophagus and possibly inflamed esophageal mucosa.[73–76] In these situations, it might be almost impossible to interpret the study, because the reader does not see a characteristic drop in impedance with reflux episodes.

SUMMARY

Diagnostic testing for GERD has evolved to include multiesophageal sites (distal, proximal, and hypopharyngeal monitoring), wireless pH, and oropharyngeal devices. The versatility of the devices has increased our ability to better understand the role of acid reflux in various disorders involving reflux of acid. Wireless pH monitoring improves patient comfort and allows monitoring for GER events over several days. Ambulatory MII-pH monitoring is another exciting diagnostic tool, which is capable of detecting more than one type of reflux and achieves higher sensitivity and specificity to detect GERD than those of endoscopy or pH-metry. It is useful in patients with either typical or atypical reflux symptoms who are refractory to PPI therapy. In this setting, MII-pH can be performed on PPI therapy to assess the efficacy of PPIs and the role of nonacid or acid reflux in persistent symptoms.

REFERENCES

1. Sarani B, Gleiber M, Evans SR. Esophageal pH monitoring, indications, and methods. J Clin Gastroenterol 2002;34(3):200–6.
2. Fuchs KH, DeMeester TR, Albertucci M. Specificity and sensitivity of objective diagnosis of gastroesophageal reflux disease. Surgery 1987;102(4):575–80.

3. Numans ME, et al. Short-term treatment with proton-pump inhibitors as a test for gastroesophageal reflux disease: a meta-analysis of diagnostic test characteristics. Ann Intern Med 2004;140(7):518–27.
4. Charbel S, Khandwala F, Vaezi MF. The role of esophageal pH monitoring in symptomatic patients on PPI therapy. Am J Gastroenterol 2005;100(2):283–9.
5. Johnson LF, DeMeester TR. Twenty-four-hour pH monitoring of the distal esophagus. A quantitative measure of gastroesophageal reflux. Am J Gastroenterol 1974;62(4):325–32.
6. Richter JE, et al. Normal 24-hr ambulatory esophageal pH values. Influence of study center, pH electrode, age, and gender. Dig Dis Sci 1992;37(6):849–56.
7. Wiener GJ, et al. Ambulatory 24-hour esophageal pH monitoring. Reproducibility and variability of pH parameters. Dig Dis Sci 1988;33(9):1127–33.
8. Johnson LF, DeMeester TR. Development of the 24-hour intraesophageal pH monitoring composite scoring system. J Clin Gastroenterol 1986;8(Suppl 1): 52–8.
9. Singh S, et al. The symptom index. Differential usefulness in suspected acid-related complaints of heartburn and chest pain. Dig Dis Sci 1993;38(8): 1402–8.
10. Breumelhof R, Smout AJ. The symptom sensitivity index: a valuable additional parameter in 24-hour esophageal pH recording. Am J Gastroenterol 1991; 86(2):160–4.
11. Weusten BL, et al. The symptom-association probability: an improved method for symptom analysis of 24-hour esophageal pH data. Gastroenterology 1994; 107(6):1741–5.
12. Taghavi SA, et al. Symptom association probability and symptom sensitivity index: preferable but still suboptimal predictors of response to high dose omeprazole. Gut 2005;54(8):1067–71.
13. Hirano I, et al. Four-day Bravo pH capsule monitoring with and without proton pump inhibitor therapy. Clin Gastroenterol Hepatol 2005;3(11):1083–8.
14. Pritchett J, Slaughter J, Vaezi MF. Is esophageal impedance monitoring detecting something new? A case-control study assessing predictive nature of non-acid reflux. Gastroenterology 2008;134(711):A101.
15. Anggiansah A, et al. Significantly reduced acid detection at 10 centimeters compared to 5 centimeters above lower esophageal sphincter in patients with acid reflux. Am J Gastroenterol 1993;88(6):842–6.
16. Vaezi MF, Richter JE. Role of acid and duodenogastroesophageal reflux in gastroesophageal reflux disease. Gastroenterology 1996;111(5):1192–9.
17. Ahmed T, Vaezi MF. The role of pH monitoring in extraesophageal gastroesophageal reflux disease. Gastrointest Endosc Clin N Am 2005;15(2):319–31.
18. Jacob P, Kahrilas PJ, Herzon G. Proximal esophageal pH-metry in patients with 'reflux laryngitis.' Gastroenterology 1991;100(2):305–10.
19. Koufman J, et al. Reflux laryngitis and its sequelae: the diagnostic role of ambulatory 24-hour pH monitoring. J Voice 1988;2:78–89.
20. Shaker R, et al. Esophagopharyngeal distribution of refluxed gastric acid in patients with reflux laryngitis. Gastroenterology 1995;109(5):1575–82.
21. Ylitalo R, Lindestad PA, Ramel S. Symptoms, laryngeal findings, and 24-hour pH monitoring in patients with suspected gastroesophago-pharyngeal reflux. Laryngoscope 2001;111(10):1735–41.
22. Oelschlager BK, et al. Laryngoscopy and pharyngeal pH are complementary in the diagnosis of gastroesophageal-laryngeal reflux. J Gastrointest Surg 2002; 6(2):189–94.

23. Vaezi MF, Schroeder PL, Richter JE. Reproducibility of proximal probe pH parameters in 24-hour ambulatory esophageal pH monitoring. Am J Gastroenterol 1997; 92(5):825–9.
24. Shaker R, et al. Intrapharyngeal distribution of gastric acid refluxate. Laryngoscope 2003;113(7):1182–91.
25. Bilgen C, et al. The comparison of an empiric proton pump inhibitor trial vs 24-hour double-probe pH monitoring in laryngopharyngeal reflux. J Laryngol Otol 2003;117(5):386–90.
26. Maldonado A, et al. Laryngopharyngeal reflux identified using a new catheter design: defining normal values and excluding artifacts. Laryngoscope 2003; 113(2):349–55.
27. Wong WM, et al. Feasibility and tolerability of transnasal/per-oral placement of the wireless pH capsule vs. traditional 24-h oesophageal pH monitoring–a randomized trial. Aliment Pharmacol Ther 2005;21(2):155–63.
28. Kahrilas PJ, et al. The effect of hiatus hernia on gastro-oesophageal junction pressure. Gut 1999;44(4):476–82.
29. Pandolfino JE, et al. Ambulatory esophageal pH monitoring using a wireless system. Am J Gastroenterol 2003;98(4):740–9.
30. Clouse R, Prakash C, Haroian L. Symptom association tests are improved by the extended ambulatory pH recording time with Bravo capsule. Gastroenterology 2003;124:A537.
31. Sifrim D, et al. Gastro-oesophageal reflux monitoring: review and consensus report on detection and definitions of acid, non-acid, and gas reflux. Gut 2004; 53(7):1024–31.
32. Vela MF, et al. Simultaneous intraesophageal impedance and pH measurement of acid and nonacid gastroesophageal reflux: effect of omeprazole. Gastroenterology 2001;120(7):1599–606.
33. Vaezi MF, Shay SS. New techniques in measuring nonacidic esophageal reflux. Semin Thorac Cardiovasc Surg 2001;13(3):255–64.
34. Sifrim D, et al. Acid, nonacid, and gas reflux in patients with gastroesophageal reflux disease during ambulatory 24-hour pH-impedance recordings. Gastroenterology 2001;120(7):1588–98.
35. Sifrim D, et al. Patterns of gas and liquid reflux during transient lower oesophageal sphincter relaxation: a study using intraluminal electrical impedance. Gut 1999;44(1):47–54.
36. Blom D, et al. Esophageal bolus transport identified by simultaneous multichannel intraluminal impedance and manofluoroscopy. Gastroenterology 2001;120:P103.
37. Silny J. Intraluminal multiple electrical impedance procedure for measurement of gastrointestinal motility. J Gastrointest Mot 1991;3:151–62.
38. Tutuian R, et al. Multichannel intraluminal impedance in esophageal function testing and gastroesophageal reflux monitoring. J Clin Gastroenterol 2003; 37(3):206–15.
39. Silny J, et al. Verification of the intraluminal multiple electrical impedance measurement for recording of gastrointestinal motility. J Gastrointest Mot 1993; 5:107–22.
40. Anandasabapathy S, Jaffin BW. Multichannel intraluminal impedance in the evaluation of patients with persistent globus on proton pump inhibitor therapy. Ann Otol Rhinol Laryngol 2006;115(8):563–70.
41. Kawamura O, et al. Physical and pH properties of gastroesophagopharyngeal refluxate: a 24-hour simultaneous ambulatory impedance and pH monitoring study. Am J Gastroenterol 2004;99(6):1000–10.

42. Weigt J, et al. Multichannel intraluminal impedance and pH-metry for investigation of symptomatic gastroesophageal reflux disease. Dig Dis 2007;25(3): 179–82.
43. Castell DO, et al. Esomeprazole (40 mg) compared with lansoprazole (30 mg) in the treatment of erosive esophagitis. Am J Gastroenterol 2002;97(3):575–83.
44. Shay S, et al. Multichannel intraluminal impedance (MII) in the evaluation of patients with persistent GERD symptoms despite proton pump inhibitors (PPI): a multicenter study. Gastroenterology 2003;124(Suppl 1):A537.
45. Shay SS, Eggli D, Johnson LF. Simultaneous esophageal pH monitoring and scintigraphy during the postprandial period in patients with severe reflux esophagitis. Dig Dis Sci 1991;36(5):558–64.
46. Sifrim D, et al. Composition of the postprandial refluxate in patients with gastroesophageal reflux disease. Am J Gastroenterol 2001;96(3):647–55.
47. Shay S, et al. Twenty-four hour ambulatory simultaneous impedance and pH monitoring: a multicenter report of normal values from 60 healthy volunteers. Am J Gastroenterol 2004;99(6):1037–43.
48. Jeske HC, et al. Preoperative administration of esomeprazole has no influence on frequency of refluxes. J Clin Anesth 2008;20(3):191–5.
49. Tutuian R, et al. Normal values for ambulatory 24-hour combined impedance-pH monitoring on acid suppressive therapy. Gastroenterology 2006;130(Suppl 2): A171.
50. Zerbib F, et al. Esophageal pH-impedance monitoring and symptom analysis in GERD: a study in patients off and on therapy. Am J Gastroenterol 2006;101(9): 1956–63.
51. Bredenoord AJ, et al. Addition of esophageal impedance monitoring to pH monitoring increases the yield of symptom association analysis in patients off PPI therapy. Am J Gastroenterol 2006;101(3):453–9.
52. Peter CS, et al. Gastroesophageal reflux and apnea of prematurity: no temporal relationship. Pediatrics 2002;109(1):8–11.
53. Rosen R, Nurko S. The importance of multichannel intraluminal impedance in the evaluation of children with persistent respiratory symptoms. Am J Gastroenterol 2004;99(12):2452–8.
54. Skopnik H, et al. Gastroesophageal reflux in infants: evaluation of a new intraluminal impedance technique. J Pediatr Gastroenterol Nutr 1996;23(5): 591–8.
55. Wenzl TG, et al. Association of apnea and nonacid gastroesophageal reflux in infants: Investigations with the intraluminal impedance technique. Pediatr Pulmonol 2001;31(2):144–9.
56. Lazenby JP, Harding SM. Chronic cough, asthma, and gastroesophageal reflux. Curr Gastroenterol Rep 2000;2(3):217–23.
57. Wenzl TG, et al. Gastroesophageal reflux and respiratory phenomena in infants: status of the intraluminal impedance technique. J Pediatr Gastroenterol Nutr 1999;28(4):423–8.
58. Richter JE. Ear, nose and throat and respiratory manifestations of gastro-esophageal reflux disease: an increasing conundrum. Eur J Gastroenterol Hepatol 2004;16(9):837–45.
59. Tack J, et al. Gastroesophageal reflux disease poorly responsive to single-dose proton pump inhibitors in patients without Barrett's esophagus: acid reflux, bile reflux, or both? Am J Gastroenterol 2004;99(6):981–8.
60. Vaezi MF. "Refractory GERD:" acid, nonacid, or not GERD? Am J Gastroenterol 2004;99(6):989–90.

61. Bajbouj M, et al. Combined pH-metry/impedance monitoring increases the diagnostic yield in patients with atypical gastroesophageal reflux symptoms. Digestion 2007;76(3–4):223–8.
62. Tamhankar AP, et al. Omeprazole does not reduce gastroesophageal reflux: new insights using multichannel intraluminal impedance technology. J Gastrointest Surg 2004;8(7):890–7 [discussion: 897–8].
63. Emerenziani S, et al. Presence of gas in the refluxate enhances reflux perception in non-erosive patients with physiological acid exposure of the oesophagus. Gut 2008;57(4):443–7.
64. Tutuian R, et al. Characteristics of symptomatic reflux episodes on acid suppressive therapy. Am J Gastroenterol 2008;103(5):1090–6.
65. Zerbib F, et al. Determinants of gastro-oesophageal reflux perception in patients with persistent symptoms despite proton pump inhibitors. Gut 2008;57(2): 156–60.
66. Mainie I, et al. Combined multichannel intraluminal impedance-pH monitoring to select patients with persistent gastro-oesophageal reflux for laparoscopic Nissen fundoplication. Br J Surg 2006;93(12):1483–7.
67. Vaezi MF, et al. Laryngeal signs and symptoms and gastroesophageal reflux disease (GERD): a critical assessment of cause and effect association. Clin Gastroenterol Hepatol 2003;1(5):333–44.
68. Park W, Vaezi MF. Is reflux laryngitis refractory to high dose PPI therapy caused by persistent acid or non-acid reflux? Gastroenterology 2005;128:M1778.
69. Swoger J, et al. Surgical fundoplication in laryngopharyngeal reflux unresponsive to aggressive acid suppression: a controlled study. Clin Gastroenterol Hepatol 2006;4(4):433–41.
70. Mainie I, et al. Acid and non-acid reflux in patients with persistent symptoms despite acid suppressive therapy: a multicentre study using combined ambulatory impedance-pH monitoring. Gut 2006;55(10):1398–402.
71. Wasko-Czopnik D, Blonski W, Paradowski L. Diagnostic difficulties during combined multichannel intraluminal impedance and pH monitoring in patients with esophagitis or Barrett's esophagus. Adv Med Sci 2007;52:196–8.
72. Domingues GR, et al. Characteristics of oesophageal bolus transport in patients with mild oesophagitis. Eur J Gastroenterol Hepatol 2005;17(3):323–32.
73. Blonski W, et al. An analysis of distal esophageal impedance in individuals with and without esophageal motility abnormalities. J Clin Gastroenterol 2008;42(7):776–81.
74. Vela MF, et al. Baclofen decreases acid and non-acid post-prandial gastro-oesophageal reflux measured by combined multichannel intraluminal impedance and pH. Aliment Pharmacol Ther 2003;17(2):243–51.
75. Conchillo JM, et al. Role of intra-oesophageal impedance monitoring in the evaluation of endoscopic gastroplication for gastro-oesophageal reflux disease. Aliment Pharmacol Ther 2007;26(1):61–8.
76. Mainie I, et al. Fundoplication eliminates chronic cough due to non-acid reflux identified by impedance pH monitoring. Thorax 2005;60(6):521–3.

Functional Heartburn: What It Is and How to Treat It

Ronnie Fass, MD

KEYWORDS

- Heartburn • Esophagus • pH testing
- Functional esophageal disorder • Proton pump inhibitor

Functional gastrointestinal disorders can affect any level of the gastrointestinal tract, from the esophagus (eg, functional dysphagia and globus sensation) to the colon and rectum (eg, functional constipation and rectal pain). Patients with these disorders are frequently seen in primary care settings as well as in tertiary referral centers. In a United States householder survey for functional gastrointestinal disorders using the Rome I diagnostic criteria, the national prevalence for one or more functional gastrointestinal disorders was estimated to be as high as 70%.[1] Forty-two percent of the responders reported at least one symptom that was attributed to the esophagus. For comparison, a similar proportion of responders (44%) reported symptoms that were related to the large bowel.

The Rome II criteria,[2] formulated in 1999, were used in a Canadian householder survey. At least one functional gastrointestinal disorder was detected in 61.7% of the 1149 responders to a mailed questionnaire. Functional disorders of the bowel were the most prevalent, diagnosed in 41.6% of the responders, whereas functional esophageal disorders were diagnosed in 28.9%.[3] The most prevalent functional esophageal disorder, detected in 22.3% of the responders, was functional heartburn. Although the symptoms of functional gastrointestinal disorders in this population-based study were significantly more prevalent in female subjects, no gender predilection was demonstrated in esophageal-related functional symptoms.[3]

As a group, functional esophageal disorders are characterized by the presence of chronic symptoms attributed to the esophagus without evidence of structural or metabolic disorder. According to the Rome III criteria, patients should experience functional esophageal disorders for at least 3 months with symptom onset at least 6 months before diagnosis (**Box 1**).[4] Nonesophageal sources for symptoms should be excluded first before esophageal causes are entertained. Gastroesophageal reflux disease (GERD) and various esophageal motility disorders may be responsible

Section of Gastroenterology, Department of Medicine, Southern Arizona VA Health Care System and University of Arizona Health Sciences Center, GI Section (1-111G-1), 3601 South. 6th Avenue, Tucson, AZ 85723–0001, USA
E-mail address: Ronnie.Fass@va.gov

Gastrointest Endoscopy Clin N Am 19 (2009) 23–33
doi:10.1016/j.giec.2008.12.002
1052-5157/08/$ – see front matter © 2009 Elsevier Inc. All rights reserved.

Box 1
Functional Esophageal Disorders (Rome III)

- Functional heartburn
- Functional chest pain of presumed esophageal origin
- Functional dysphagia
- Globus

---

for the spectrum of functional esophageal-related symptoms. Hence, it is imperative that these conditions be ruled out before a diagnosis of a functional esophageal disorder is established. Rome III also removed rumination syndrome from the functional esophageal disorder group and added it to the functional gastroduodenal disorders. Although the Rome project attempts to repeatedly update the diagnostic criteria of the different functional bowel disorders, the relatively high frequency (approximately every 5 years) of the meetings that are commonly associated with changes in diagnostic criteria may render past and ongoing studies in this field obsolete.

Although benign in nature, functional gastrointestinal disorders cause considerable impairment in quality of life and result in a significant economic burden on the health care system.[5–8] Additionally, the obscure pathophysiologic basis of these conditions commonly results in frustration for both patients and physicians. Moreover, therapies are mainly empiric in nature and, in many cases, of limited value.

DEFINITION

Classic GERD symptoms (eg, heartburn and acid regurgitation) in the presence of a normal esophageal mucosa have been used to define nonerosive reflux disease (NERD).[9] Fass and colleagues[10] suggested an alternative definition offering a more pathophysiologic perspective; NERD is defined as classic GERD symptoms caused by gastroesophageal reflux in the absence of visible esophageal mucosal injury. This definition emphasizes the relationship between gastroesophageal reflux (acid and nonacid) and classic GERD symptoms regardless of whether the total time with pH less than 4 is abnormal or within the normal range. Additionally, it excludes those patients with heartburn from non–reflux-related stimuli (eg, motor event).

Early studies originating from tertiary referral centers suggested that approximately half of the patients presenting with typical reflux-related symptoms had erosive esophagitis on upper endoscopy. However, later studies that were performed in the community revealed that up to 70% of the GERD patients have NERD.[10]

Studies have demonstrated that patients with NERD are a heterogeneous group. Further subcategorization of NERD relies primarily on the results of 24-hour esophageal pH monitoring. Approximately half of the patients who fall under the category of NERD have normal esophageal acid exposure during 24-hour esophageal pH monitoring.[11] The Rome II Committee for Functional Esophageal Disorders considered these patients as having functional heartburn. The latter was defined as an episodic retrosternal burning in the absence of pathologic gastroesophageal reflux or pathology-based motility disorders.[4] Thus, according to Rome II criteria, patients with functional heartburn demonstrate normal esophageal mucosa on endoscopy as well as esophageal acid exposure within the normal range.[2] Furthermore, these patients were divided into 2 main groups: those who demonstrated a close relationship between their symptoms and acid reflux events (the hypersensitive group) and those who reported heartburn symptoms that were not related to acid reflux events.

The Rome III Committee for Functional Esophageal Disorders redefined functional heartburn primarily by excluding the hypersensitive group and incorporating them with NERD (**Box 2**).[4] In addition, those who are left under the category of functional heartburn should also demonstrate lack of response to a full course of proton pump inhibitor (PPI) treatment. PPI responders are also excluded from the functional heartburn group. It is unclear from Rome III criteria if patients have to demonstrate lack of symptomatic response to PPI once daily or to higher doses.

Functional bowel disorders are commonly characterized by increased visceral sensitivity to low-intensity stimuli. Functional heartburn patients who are sensitive to physiologic amounts of acid fulfill these criteria, regardless of whether they are responsive to antireflux treatment. Furthermore, to meet the new Rome III criteria for functional heartburn, patients will have to go through one course of treatment with standard-dose PPI once daily (2 months), and if they are still nonresponders, another 2 months of treatment course should be followed with PPI twice daily. As a result, the new Rome III criteria for functional heartburn are likely to make studies in functional heartburn much more labor intensive and costly. Presently, there are almost no studies on functional heartburn using Rome III criteria. Consequently, the information presented here is solely based on Rome II criteria for functional heartburn.

EPIDEMIOLOGY

Given that patients with heartburn and normal esophageal mucosa account for up to 70% of heartburn patients in the community, functional heartburn appears to be a very common phenomenon affecting about 50% of the subjects. In approximately 40% of the patients with functional heartburn (based on Rome II criteria), a close relationship can be demonstrated between their symptoms and acid reflux events (hypersensitive esophagus). The remaining 60% of patients with functional heartburn lack any temporal relationship between their symptoms and esophageal acid reflux events. Symptom generation in these patients is likely not related to acid and may be the consequence of bile reflux, alkaline reflux, various motor events (eg, volume distention), or other unidentified intraesophageal stimuli.

The demographics of patients with functional heartburn have been scarcely studied. When compared with patients with NERD, those with functional heartburn have the same female predominance and mean age (**Table 1**).[12] The range of *Helicobacter pylori* infection is between 30% and 45%, and hiatal hernia is very uncommon (20%). There is no difference in symptom characteristics between functional heartburn and NERD except for a longer history of heartburn in patients with functional heartburn. Concomitant functional bowel or other gastrointestinal (GI) disorders as well

---

Box 2
Diagnostic criteria (Rome III) for functional heartburn

Must include all of the following:

- Burning retrosternal discomfort or pain
- Absence of evidence that gastroesophageal reflux is the cause of the symptom
- Absence of histopathology-based esophageal motility disorders

Criteria fulfilled for the last 3 months with symptom onset at least 6 months before diagnosis

Table 1
Characteristics of functional heartburn patients compared with NERD patients (using Rome II criteria)

	FH	NERD	P
Gender	F > M	F > M	NS
Mean age	46 y	43 y	NS
H. pylori positive	30%–45%	30%–50%	NS
Hiatal hernia	20%	20%	NS
History of heartburn (y)	7.5	3.5	<.05
Chest pain episodes	Once a week	Once a month	<.05
Symptom severity	Similar	Similar	NS
Symptom frequency	Similar	Similar	NS
Concomitant FBD	Similar	Similar	NS
Concomitant other GI disorders	Similar	Similar	NS
HRQOL (SF-30)	Similar	Similar	NS

Abbreviations: FBD–functional bowel disease; F, female; FH, functional heartburn; GI, gastrointestinal; HRQOL, health-related quality of life; M, male; NERD, nonerosive reflux disease; NS, not significant; SF-30, short-form 36-item questionnaire.

as reported quality of life are not different between the two disorders. History of chest pain episodes is more common in functional heartburn than in NERD patients. This may suggest that other functional esophageal disorders are common in functional heartburn patients. The psychological profile of functional heartburn patients is similar to that of NERD patients except for an increase in reports of somatization (**Fig. 1**).

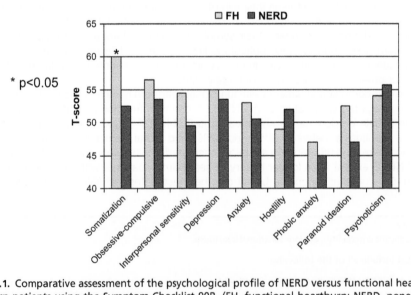

Fig. 1. Comparative assessment of the psychological profile of NERD versus functional heartburn patients using the Symptom Checklist-90R. (FH, functional heartburn; NERD, nonerosive reflux disease.) (*From* Shapiro M, Green C, Bautista J, et al. Functional heartburn patients demonstrate traits of functional bowel disorder but lack a uniform increase of chemoreceptor sensitivity to acid. Am J Gastroenterol 2006;101(5):1084–91; with permission.)

ETIOLOGY

Repeated studies in patients with functional heartburn who use either esophageal balloon distention or electrical stimulation have consistently demonstrated a lower perception threshold for pain compared with that in patients with other presentations of GERD.[13] Furthermore, objective neurophysiologic measures of esophageal evoked potential latency revealed that functional heartburn patients achieve equivalent latency and amplitude responses with reduced afferent input, suggesting heightened esophageal sensitivity.[14] By contrast, stimulus response functions to acid in patients with functional heartburn gave mixed results. Rodriguez-Stanley and colleagues[15] reported that 90% of patients with functional heartburn experienced abnormal responses to esophageal balloon distention, intraesophageal acid perfusion (Bernstein test), or both. Thoua and colleagues[16] have demonstrated increased esophageal hypersensitivity in patients with functional heartburn compared with that in patients with NERD or erosive esophagitis. On the other hand, Shapiro and colleagues[12] demonstrated a higher mean value for time to heartburn symptoms and lower mean values for intensity and acid perfusion sensitivity score than those in patients with NERD and abnormal pH testing. Additionally, a quarter of patients with functional heartburn had a negative acid perfusion test. This study further supports the hypothesis that functional heartburn is composed from a heterogeneous group of patients.

Increased mechanoreceptor sensitivity to balloon distention seems to be a general phenomenon in functional heartburn compared with only a subset of patients who show increased chemoreceptor sensitivity to acid. Overall, it seems that esophageal hypersensitivity is an important mechanism in functional heartburn. Central neural mechanisms,[17,18] such as psychological comorbidity (anxiety, stress, and depression), can modulate esophageal perception and cause patients to perceive low-intensity esophageal stimuli as being painful. However, it is still unclear what role these central factors play in symptom generation of patients with functional heartburn. Yang and colleagues[19] have demonstrated that cortical evoked potential responses resulting from esophageal distention and acid perfusion were greater in patients with functional heartburn than in controls. The authors suggested that visceral neural pathway dysfunction and/or alteration in central processing may precipitate esophageal hypersensitivity in functional heartburn patients.[19]

Frazzoni and colleagues[20] evaluated patients with different phenotypic presentations of GERD and compared them with functional heartburn patients and normal controls. Patients with functional heartburn did not differ from normal controls in their distal esophageal acid exposure profile, prevalence of hiatal hernia, distal esophageal amplitude contractions, and lower esophageal sphincter basal pressure. This study promotes the concept that mechanisms other than reflux are likely to have an important role in symptom generation of patients with functional heartburn. Martinez and colleagues[11] demonstrated that patients with NERD and an abnormal pH test were more likely to have a symptom index greater than 75% than were functional heartburn patients (69.5% versus 10.5%, $P = .0001$).[11] In the functional heartburn group, those patients with a negative symptom index reported having heartburn at a pH less than four only 12.7% of the time compared with 70.7% of the time in those with a positive symptom index, despite a similar mean number of heartburn episodes.[11]

Several local factors have been suggested to play an important role in symptom generation of patients with functional heartburn. Cicala and colleagues[21] have demonstrated that patients with functional heartburn (per Rome II criteria) have the highest proximal acid exposure that is associated with heartburn compared with those with NERD or erosive esophagitis.[21] Proximal migration of esophageal acid exposure has been shown to be an important factor in symptom generation of GERD patients, but more specifically in those with functional heartburn (**Fig. 2**).[16,22,23] Dilated intercellular spaces (DIS), which are commonly seen in GERD patients and are currently considered essential for acid to access sensory afferents that are located in the esophageal mucosa, have also been observed in patients with functional heartburn (**Fig. 3**).[24] pH-impedance studies did not find any difference in the extent of weakly acidic reflux between functional heartburn and the different GERD groups.[23,25] However, the presence of gas in the refluxate appears to enhance reflux perception in functional heartburn patients.[25]

Oxidative DNA damage to the epithelial cells of the esophagus has been shown to occur after acid exposure. A subset of functional heartburn patients demonstrate this immunohistochemical abnormality.[26] It is yet to be determined whether these are primarily hypersensitive esophagus patients.

Shapiro and colleagues[12] have suggested that functional heartburn patients demonstrate traits of a functional bowel disorder. The authors have shown increased reports of chest pain and somatization by patients as well as alteration in autonomic function.

DIAGNOSIS

Establishing the diagnosis of functional heartburn requires two invasive procedures: upper endoscopy and 24-hour esophageal pH monitoring.[13] The yield of random distal esophageal biopsies to assess the presence of typical GERD-related histopathologic findings and thus improve diagnosis of GERD in patients with functional heartburn is very low. Histologic evidence of acid-related mucosal injury can be found in less than 10% of the patients.[27] Consequently, the role of upper endoscopy is limited to exclusion of esophageal mucosal involvement.

Esophageal pH monitoring for 24 hours allows identification of patients with either normal or abnormal distal esophageal acid exposure and determination of the temporal relationship between their symptoms and acid reflux events. The

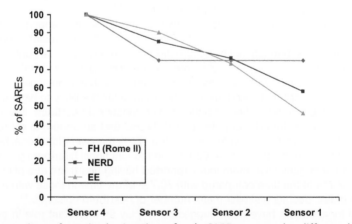

Fig. 2. Comparison of proximal migration of only SAREs among the different heartburn groups. (EE–erosive esophagitis; FH, functional heartburn; NERD, nonerosive reflux disease; SAREs, sensed acid reflux events.) (*From* Schey R, Shapiro M, Navarro-Rodriguez T, et al. Comparison of the different characteristics of sensed reflux events among the different heartburn groups. J Clin Gastroenterol 2008 Sep 12 [Epub ahead of print]; with permission.)

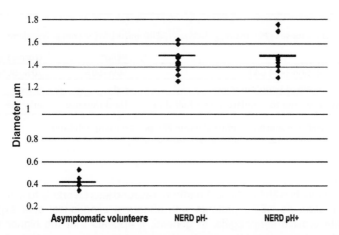

Fig. 3. Comparison of mean intercellular space diameters of esophageal epithelium among asymptomatic volunteers, NERD (NERD pH+), and functional heartburn (NERD pH-)groups. (*From* Caviglia R, Ribolsi M, Maggiano N, et al. Dilated intercellular spaces of esophageal epithelium in nonerosive reflux disease patients with physiologic esophageal acid exposure. Am J Gastroenterol 2005;100(3):543–8; with permission.)

introduction of the Bravo pH monitoring system (Medtronic, North Shoreview, Minnesota), a catheter-free approach for ambulatory esophageal pH monitoring, raised the hopes of improved tolerability of the pH test. Surprisingly, patients with functional heartburn were more likely to report retrosternal discomfort after placement of the Bravo pH capsule.[28] This finding further supports the importance of esophageal hyperalgesia as an underlying mechanism for symptom generation in patients with functional heartburn.

FUNCTIONAL HEARTBURN AND REFRACTORY GERD

It has been estimated that between 10% and 40% of patients with GERD fail to respond symptomatically, either partially or completely, to a standard dose PPI.[29–32] During a period of only 7 years (1997–2004), there was an increase of almost 50% in the usage of at least double-dose PPI in patients with GERD.[33] Additionally, it appears that less than 50% of the GERD patients are satisfied with their medical treatment, and only 58% of those receiving PPI report a high level of satisfaction with their therapy.[31]

Studies have consistently demonstrated that NERD patients have a lower symptomatic response rate to PPI than that in patients with erosive esophagitis.[33] **Table 2** demonstrates the striking differences in various symptomatic response parameters between the two patient groups. An important reason for such a wide discrepancy in symptom reports is the repeated inclusion of functional heartburn patients in almost all of the NERD-related therapeutic studies. Because exclusion of these patients from the NERD group requires pH testing, many of the investigators elected not to subject the patients to such an invasive test and consequently included the functional heartburn patients in the NERD group.

Studies evaluating patients who did not respond to PPI twice daily demonstrated that up to 58% of them have functional heartburn.[34,35] Thus, functional heartburn is the most common cause for failure of PPI treatment.

	NERD[a]	Erosive Esophagitis
Symptom resolution (at 4 wk)	50%–60%	70%–80%
Lag time to sustained symptom relief	6 d	4–5 d
Symptomatic response to standard versus half dose	No difference	Increase

Abbreviations: NERD, nonerosive reflux disease; PPI, proton pump inhibitor.
[a] NERD includes patients with functional heartburn.

TREATMENT

As a group, patients with functional heartburn respond less favorably to acid-suppressive therapy than do NERD patients with abnormal esophageal acid exposure or patients with erosive esophagitis. In general, it appears that the higher the distal esophageal acid exposure, the greater the symptom response rate to a standard dose of PPI in patients with NERD.[36] Approximately 50% of patients with functional heartburn failed treatment with a standard dose of PPI.[36] Several studies of patients with functional heartburn treated with a PPI have demonstrated that a double or even triple dose is needed to improve symptom response (37%–60%).[37–39] Patients with a hypersensitive esophagus are more likely to respond to PPI treatment. How high one can raise the PPI dose and still improve symptoms or increase the number of responders is still to be elucidated. Nevertheless, PPIs remain the best initial treatment, albeit a limited one, for patients with functional heartburn. A study in 2008 by Aanen and colleagues[40] demonstrated that response to PPI is dependent on the symptom–reflux association. Functional heartburn patients with a positive symptom association probability were more likely to respond to PPI treatment than subjects with no association between their symptoms and acid reflux events.[40]

Patients with functional heartburn who do not respond to PPI treatment are likely to experience heartburn as a result of various non–acid-related stimuli. Successful therapeutic strategies for this group of patients must address the underlying mechanism responsible for their symptoms. For example, motor events, such as sustained contractions of the esophageal longitudinal muscle, have been suggested as the motor corollary of heartburn.[41] These underlying mechanisms have led some experts to suggest that smooth-muscle relaxants (eg, calcium channel blockers and nitrates) may have a role in the treatment of functional heartburn patients with non–reflux-related stimuli.[42] No data are available to support this hypothesis.

Other investigators have suggested pain modulators for the treatment of patients with functional heartburn who have failed PPI therapy. TCAs, trazodone, and selective serotonin reuptake inhibitors have shown efficacy in other functional esophageal disorders, including noncardiac chest pain.[43,44] Although the use of antidepressants is highly attractive, studies demonstrating their efficacy in functional heartburn patients are still lacking. Histamine 2 receptor antagonists have been shown to modulate esophageal acid sensitivity in patients with functional heartburn.[45] Tegaserod, a partial 5-hydroxytryptamine 4 agonist, has been shown to improve both chemo- and mechanoreceptor sensitivity to acid perfusion and balloon distention, respectively.[46] Additionally, 2 weeks of tegaserod 6 mg twice daily markedly improved patients' heartburn and other upper GI tract–related symptoms compared with placebo.

In summary, the diagnosis of functional heartburn is still dependent on upper endoscopy and pH testing. PPIs should be the first line of therapy because they are beneficial for a subset of patients with a hypersensitive esophagus. However, for most patients with functional heartburn, pain modulators are likely to provide symptom relief.[13]

REFERENCES

1. Drossman DA, Li Z, Andruzzi E, et al. U.S. householder survey of functional gastrointestinal disorders: prevalence, sociodemography, and health impact. Dig Dis Sci 1993;38:1569–80.
2. Drossman DA, Crazziari R, Talley NJ, the Rome II Multinational Working Teams. Rome II: the Functional Gastrointestinal Disorders. Diagnosis, Pathophysiology and Treatment: a Multinational Consensus. 2nd edition. Drossman DA, Corazziari E, Talley J, et al, editors. McLean (VA): Degnon Associates; 2000.
3. Thompson WG, Irvine EJ, Pare P, et al. Functional gastrointestinal disorders in Canada: first population-based survey using Rome II criteria with suggestions for improving the questionnaire. Dig Dis Sci 2002;47:225–35.
4. Drossman DA, editor. Rome III: The functional gastrointestinal disorders. 3rd edition. McLean (VA): Degnon Associates, Inc; 2006.
5. Akehurst RL, Brazier JE, Mathers N, et al. Health-related quality of life and cost impact of irritable bowel syndrome in a UK primary care setting. Pharmacoeconomics 2002;20:455–62.
6. Koloski NA, Talley NJ, Boyce PM. The impact of functional gastrointestinal disorders on quality of life. Am J Gastroenterol 2000;95:67–71.
7. Badia X, Mearin F, Balboa A, et al. Burden of illness in irritable bowel syndrome comparing Rome I and Rome II criteria. Pharmacoeconomics 2002;20:749–58.
8. El-Serag HB, Olden K, Bjorkman D. Health-related quality of life among persons with irritable bowel syndrome: a systematic review. Aliment Pharmacol Ther 2002; 16:1171–85.
9. Dent J, Brun J, Fendrick AM, et al. An evidence-based appraisal of reflux disease management: the Genval Workshop Report. Gut 1999;44(Suppl 2):S1–16.
10. Fass R, Fennerty MB, Vakil N. Nonerosive reflux disease: current concepts and dilemmas. Am J Gastroenterol 2001;96:303–14.
11. Martinez SD, Malagon IB, Garewal HS, et al. Non-erosive reflux disease (NERD): acid reflux and symptom patterns. Aliment Pharmacol Ther 2003;17:537–45.
12. Shapiro M, Green C, Bautista JM, et al. Functional heartburn patients demonstrate traits of functional bowel disorder but lack a uniform increase of chemoreceptor sensitivity to acid. Am J Gastroenterol 2006;101:1084–91.
13. Fass R, Tougas G. Functional heartburn: the stimulus, the pain and the brain. Gut 2002;51:885–92.
14. Hobson AR, Furlong PL, Aziz Q, et al. Oesophageal afferent pathway sensitivity in non-erosive reflux disease. Neurogastroenterol Motil 2008;20:877–83.
15. Rodriguez-Stanley S, Robinson M, Earnest DL, et al. Esophageal hypersensitivity may be a major cause of heartburn. Am J Gastroenterol 1999;94:628–31.
16. Thoua NM, Khoo D, Kalantzis C, et al. Acid-related oesophageal sensitivity, not dysmotility, differentiates subgroups of patients with non-erosive reflux disease. Aliment Pharmacol Ther 2008;27(5):396–403.
17. Siddiqui A, Rodriguez-Stanley S, Zubaidi S, et al. Esophageal visceral sensitivity to bile salts in patients with functional heartburn and in healthy control subjects. Dig Dis Sci 2005;50:81–5.
18. Trimble KS, Pryde A, Heading RC. Lowered oesophageal sensory thresholds in patients with symptomatic but not excess gastro-oesophageal reflux: evidence for a spectrum of visceral sensitivity in GORD. Gut 1995;37:7–12.

19. Yang M, Li Z-S, Xu X-R, et al. Characterization of cortical potentials evoked by oesophageal balloon distention and acid perfusion in patients with functional heartburn. Neurogastroenterol Motil 2006;18(4):292–9.
20. Frazzoni M, De Micheli E, Zentilin P, et al. Pathophysiological characteristics of patients with non-erosive reflux disease differ from those of patients with functional heartburn. Aliment Pharmacol Ther 2004;20:81–8.
21. Cicala M, Emerenziani S, Caviglia R, et al. Intra-oesophageal distribution and perception of acid reflux in patients with non-erosive gastro-oesophageal reflux disease. Aliment Pharmacol Ther 2003;18(6):605–13.
22. Schey R, Shapiro M, Navarro-Rodriguez T, et al. Comparison of the different characteristics of sensed reflux events among the different heartburn group. J Clin Gastroenterol 2008 [Epub ahead of print].
23. Bredenoord AJ, Weusten BL, Timmer R, et al. Characteristics of gastroesophageal reflux in symptomatic patients with and without excessive esophageal acid exposure. Am J Gastroenterol 2006;101(11):2470–5.
24. Caviglia R, Ribolsi M, Maggiano N, et al. Dilated intercellular spaces of esophageal epithelium in nonerosive reflux disease patients with physiological esophageal acid exposure. Am J Gastroenterol 2005;100(3):543–8.
25. Emerenziani S, Sifrim D, Habib FI, et al. Presence of gas in the refluxate enhances reflux perception in non-erosive patients with physiological acid exposure of the oesophagus. Gut 2008;57(4):443–7.
26. Liu L, Ergun G, Ertan A, et al. Detection of oxidative DNA damage in oesophageal biopsies of patients with reflux symptoms and normal pH monitoring. Aliment Pharmacol Ther 2003;18(7):693–8.
27. Schindlbeck NE, Wiebecke B, Klauser AG, et al. Diagnostic value of histology in non-erosive gastro-oesophageal reflux disease. Gut 1996;39:151–4.
28. Lee Y-C, Wang H-P, Chiu H-M, et al. Patients with functional heartburn are more likely to report retrosternal discomfort during wireless pH monitoring. Gastrointest Endosc 2005;62(6):834–41.
29. Inadomi JM, McIntyre L, Bernard L, et al. Step-down from multiple- to single-dose proton pump inhibitors (PPIs): a prospective study of patients with heartburn or acid regurgitation completely relieved with PPIs. Am J Gastroenterol 2003; 98(9):1940–4.
30. Carlsson R, Dent J, Watts R, et al. Gastro-oesophageal reflux disease in primary care: an international study of different treatment strategies with omeprazole. International GORD Study Group. Eur J Gastroenterol Hepatol 1998;10(2):119–24.
31. Crawley JA, Schmitt CM. How satisfied are chronic heartburn sufferers with their prescription medications? Results of the patient unmet needs study. J Clin Outcomes Manag 2000;7:29–34.
32. Gallup Organization. The 2000 Gallup Study of Consumers' Use of Stomach Relief Products. Princeton (NJ): Gallup Organization; 2000.
33. Dean BB, Gano AD Jr, Knight K, et al. Effectiveness of proton pump inhibitors in nonerosive reflux disease. Clin Gastroenterol Hepatol 2004;2:656–64.
34. Mainie I, Tutuian R, Shay S, et al. Acid and non-acid reflux in patients with persistent symptoms despite acid suppressive therapy: a multicentre study using combined ambulatory impedance-pH monitoring. Gut 2006;55(10):1398–402.
35. Sharma N, Agrawal A, Freeman J, et al. An Analysis of Persistent symptoms in acid-suppressed patients undergoing impedance-pH monitoring. Clin Gastroenterol Hepatol 2008;6(5):521–4.

36. Lind T, Havelund T, Carlsson R, et al. Heartburn without oesophagitis: efficacy of omeprazole therapy and features determining therapeutic response. Scand J Gastroenterol 1997;32:974–9.
37. Schenk BE, Kuipers EJ, Klinkenberg-Knol E, et al. Omeprazole as a diagnostic tool in gastroesophageal reflux disease. Am J Gastroenterol 1997;92:1997–2000.
38. Fass R, Ofman JJ, Gralnek IM, et al. Clinical and economic assessment of the omeprazole test in patients with symptoms suggestive of gastroesophageal reflux disease. Arch Intern Med 1999;150:2161–8.
39. Watson R, Tham T, Johnston B, et al. Double blind cross-over placebo controlled study of omeprazole in the treatment of patients with reflux symptoms. Gut 1997; 40:587–90.
40. Aanen MC, Weusten BLAM, Numans ME, et al. Effect of proton-pump inhibitor treatment on symptoms and quality of life in GERD patients depends on the symptom-reflux association. J Clin Gastroenterol 2008;42(5):441–7.
41. Pehlivanov N, Liu J, Mittal RK. Sustained esophageal contraction: a motor correlate of heartburn symptom. Am J Physiol Gastrointest Liver Physiol 2001;281: G743–51.
42. Tack J, Janssens J. Functional heartburn. Curr Treat Options Gastroenterol 2002; 5:251–8.
43. Clouse RE, Lustman PJ, Eckert TC, et al. Low-dose trazodone for symptomatic patients with esophageal contraction abnormalities: a double-blind, placebo-controlled trial. Gastroenterol 1987;92:1027–36.
44. Cannon RO III, Quyyumi AA, Mincemoyer R, et al. Imipramine in patients with chest pain despite normal coronary angiograms. N Engl J Med 1994;330:1411–7.
45. Rodriguez-Stanley S, Ciociola AA, Zubaidi S, et al. A single dose of ranitidine 150 mg modulates oesophageal acid sensitivity in patients with functional heartburn. Aliment Pharmacol Ther 2004;20:975–82.
46. Rodriguez-Stanley S, Zubaidi S, Proskin HM, et al. Effect of tegaserod on esophageal pain threshold, regurgitation, and symptom relief in patients with functional heartburn and mechanical sensitivity. Clin Gastroenterol Hepatol 2006;4(4): 442–50.

Surgical Therapy for Gastroesophageal Reflux Disease: Indications, Evaluation, and Procedures

C. Daniel Smith, MD

KEYWORDS

- Gastroesophageal reflux • GERD • Antireflux surgery
- Fundoplication

Antireflux surgery (ARS) is an appropriate and effective treatment for patients with gastroesophageal reflux disease (GERD) refractory to medical management, those on life-long acid suppression, or patients suffering from side effects of medical management. Over the past two decades, the procedures have evolved from predominantly open thoracic approaches to now a predominantly laparoscopic abdominal approach, with similar, if not better outcomes. More recently, endolumenal approaches have evolved and yet even less invasive procedures for GERD. The success of antireflux procedures in managing GERD lies largely in an understanding of GERD and its diagnosis, proper patient selection, sound operative technique, and postprocedure management. As our understanding of ARS has evolved and newer approaches and techniques have evolved, it is also important to understand how these newer procedures fit in the spectrum of options for GERD management.

GERD

GERD is defined as the failure of the antireflux barrier, allowing abnormal reflux of gastric contents into the esophagus.[1,2] It is a mechanical disorder that is caused by a defective lower esophageal sphincter (LES), a gastric emptying disorder, or failed esophageal peristalsis. These abnormalities result in a spectrum of diseases ranging from the symptom of "heartburn" to esophageal tissue damage with subsequent complications of stricture, bleeding, or metaplastic mucosal changes (Barrett's changes). As diagnostic tools have become more widely available and applied, a host of extra-esophageal manifestations of GERD are also being increasingly identified (eg, asthma, laryngitis, dental breakdown).[3,4]

Department of Surgery, Mayo Clinic, 4500 San Pablo Road, Jacksonville, FL 32224, USA
E-mail address: smith.c.daniel@mayo.edu

Gastrointest Endoscopy Clin N Am 19 (2009) 35–48
doi:10.1016/j.giec.2008.12.007
1052-5157/08/$ – see front matter © 2009 Elsevier Inc. All rights reserved.

GERD is an extremely common condition accounting for nearly 75% of all esophageal pathology. Nearly 44% of Americans experience monthly heartburn and 18% of these individuals use nonprescription medication directed against GERD. With a prevalence of nearly 19 million cases per year with an associated total cost of care of $9.8 billion in the United States, GERD is clearly a significant public health concern.[5]

There is considerable debate regarding optimal treatment of GERD. With a significant number of Americans experiencing daily heartburn and the impact this condition has on an individual's quality of life, it is no surprise that there is a tremendous amount of interest and effort going into understanding this condition and establishing effective treatment algorithms.

Medical therapy is the first line of management for GERD (**Fig. 1**). Although esophagitis will heal in approximately 90% of cases with intensive medical therapy, medical management does not address the condition's mechanical etiology; thus, symptoms recur in more than 80% of cases within 1 year of drug withdrawal.[6,7] Additionally, although medical therapy may effectively treat the acid-induced symptoms of GERD, esophageal mucosal injury may continue due to ongoing alkaline reflux. Finally, for many patients, medical therapy may be required for the rest of their lives. The expense and psychological burden of a lifetime of medication dependence, undesirable lifestyle changes, uncertainty as to the long-term effects of some newer medications, and the potential for persistent mucosal changes despite symptomatic control all make surgical treatment of GERD an attractive option.

Historically, ARS was recommended only for patients with refractory or complicated gastroesophageal reflux.[8,9] Through the early 1990s several major developments have changed our thinking regarding the long-term management of patients with GERD. First, the introduction of proton pump inhibitors (PPIs) has provided a truly effective medical therapy for GERD. Therefore, very few patients have "refractory" GERD. Second, laparoscopic surgery became available, thereby significantly changing the morbidity and recovery following an antireflux procedure. Third, the widespread availability and use of ambulatory pH monitoring and esophageal motility testing have dramatically improved our ability to recognize true GERD and select patients for

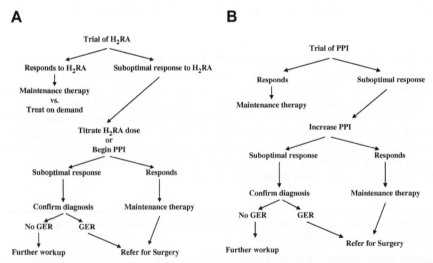

Fig. 1. Management algorithm for treatment of uncomplicated (*A*) and complicated (*B*) gastroesophageal reflux (based on endoscopic findings). H$_2$RA, H$_2$ receptor antagonist.

long-term therapy. Finally, we have realized that patients with GERD have a greatly impaired quality of life, which normalizes with successful treatment.[10]

With this, the management goals of GERD have changed. Rather than focusing therapy only on *controlling* symptoms, modern treatment of GERD aims to *eliminate* symptoms, improve a patient's quality of life, and institute a lifelong plan for management. Surgical correction of the anatomically deficient antireflux barrier is a very appealing option when trying to achieve these goals in the management of GERD.

PATIENT SELECTION FOR ARS

Selecting an appropriate patient for any antireflux procedure requires confirming the diagnosis of GERD and searching for any associated conditions that might alter one's surgical approach or options. For example, a patient with a hiatal hernia may not be a candidate for an endolumenal approach (see Endolumenal Antireflux Surgery below), or a patient with impaired esophageal clearance should be considered for a partial fundoplication rather than a full fundoplication. Understanding this, diagnosis and preoperative evaluation are critical to the success of ARS.

The clinical diagnosis of GERD is fairly straightforward if the patient reports the *typical* symptoms of heartburn or regurgitation that is readily relieved after ingesting antacids. Many patients with this classic presentation will have been treated by their primary care physician with an empirical trial of H_2 blockers or PPI, and resolution of symptoms with such treatment may be diagnostically helpful. In fact, one should be very suspicious of the diagnosis of GERD in any patient who reports no improvement in symptoms with any antisecretory regimen or in patients with *atypical* or extraesophageal symptoms such as hoarseness, chronic cough, or asthma.

Recently it has been appreciated that chest pain, asthma, laryngitis, recurrent pulmonary infections, chronic cough, and hoarseness may be associated with reflux, and this association is leading to increasing numbers of patients with these atypical GERD symptoms to be evaluated for reflux. As many as 80% of patients with asthma have endoscopic evidence of GERD,[11] and 50% of patients in whom a cardiac cause of chest pain has been excluded have acid reflux as a cause of their pain. Otolaryngologists are beginning to make primary referrals for the treatment of GERD based on chronic laryngitis and evidence of acid-induced vocal cord damage, and dentists are identifying dental damage from chronic acid reflux.

An objective diagnosis of GERD is mandatory before offering an antireflux operation, and although a barium swallow is often the first test obtained in patients suspected of having GERD, an esophagogastroduodenoscopy (EGD) is necessary in all GERD patients. Not only can an EGD confirm the diagnosis of GERD but it can also rule out other conditions such as malignancy, stricture, Barrett's esophagus, or eosinophilic esophagitis. During EGD, an esophageal mucosal biopsy should be obtained to confirm esophagitis, and esophageal length and the presence of a hiatal hernia or stricture should be assessed. If during EGD esophagitis is seen and histologically confirmed, no other tests beyond EGD are necessary to diagnose GERD. However, since most patients are already being empirically treated for GERD with PPIs, in many patients the EGD will be normal. When the diagnosis cannot be confirmed during EGD, esophageal pH testing is necessary to objectively establish the diagnosis of GERD.

The most critical aspects of patient selection is not only objective confirmation of the diagnosis but also identifying those who have conditions associated with GERD that may require special consideration. Specifically, those with associated esophageal motor disorders identified by esophageal motility testing, a shortened esophagus, or associated delayed gastric emptying may require a tailored approach to GERD. Barrett's esophagus is addressed separately below. Esophageal body dysfunction (body pressure <30 mm Hg or less than 60% peristalsis with wet swallows) may require a partial fundoplication, a shortened esophagus may require extensive mediastinal dissection to establish adequate esophageal length or a lengthening procedure, and delayed gastric emptying may require temporary postoperative gastric decompression or a drainage procedure (eg, pyloroplasty). Failure to recognize these associated problems and surgeon-derived anecdotal "modifications" to proven techniques have led to increasing numbers of patients "failing" laparoscopic ARS.[12,13]

With a thorough understanding of GERD, its associated conditions, and the various objective assessments available today, one should be able to stratify patients to select the best patient for surgery. For example, the ideal patient for ARS is one who has classic symptoms of GERD with heartburn and regurgitation as dominant symptoms, solid objective confirmation of the diagnosis, a good response to PPI therapy, and has no other confounding conditions such as Barrett's esophagus or impaired esophageal clearance. In this setting, 90%–95% of patients who have a well-done ARS will have a good outcome. In contrast, the patient who has primarily atypical symptoms, such as chronic cough or hoarseness, minimal to no improvement with PPIs, softer data to support the diagnosis of GERD (eg, no acid reflux but impedance pH showing non-acid reflux), or delayed gastric emptying or impaired esophageal clearance, will have a compromised outcome with surgery. With this atypical presentation, only 75%–85% of patients will have good symptom response to surgery, and although many will achieve objective control of their acid reflux with surgery (ie, improvement in esophageal acid exposure), many will continue to have their preoperative symptoms and will be very unhappy to have undergone an operation without relief.

PRINCIPLES AND TECHNIQUE OF ARS

The goal of ARS is to establish effective LES pressure. To realize this goal, most surgeons believe it necessary to position the LES within the abdomen where the sphincter is under positive (intra-abdominal) pressure and to close any associated hiatal defect.[14] To accomplish this, various safe and effective surgical techniques have been developed. In the last 10 years, advances in laparoscopic technology and technique have nearly eliminated open ARS. The laparoscopic techniques reproduce those in their open-surgery counterparts while eliminating the morbidity of an upper midline laparotomy incision.[15] Open antireflux operations remain indicated when the laparoscopic technique is not available or is contraindicated. Contraindications to laparoscopic ARS include uncorrectable coagulopathy, severe chronic obstructive pulmonary disease and first trimester pregnancy. Previous upper abdominal operation, and in particular prior open ARS, is a relative contraindication to a laparoscopic approach and should only be undertaken by very experienced laparoscopic surgeons.

The laparoscopic Nissen fundoplication has emerged as the most widely accepted and applied antireflux operation (**Fig. 2**).[16–21] In many centers, it is the antireflux procedure of choice in patients with normal esophageal body peristalsis. Key elements of the procedure include the following:

1. Complete dissection of the esophageal hiatus and both crura
2. Mobilization of the gastric fundus by dividing the short gastric vessels
3. Closure of the associated hiatal defect

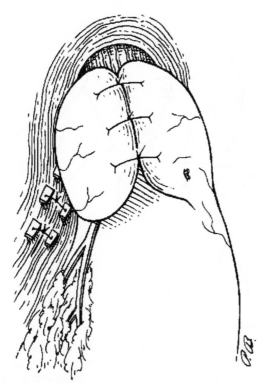

Fig. 2. Depiction of Nissen 360° fundoplication.

4. Creation of a tensionless 360° gastric wrap at the distal esophagus around a 50- to 60-F intraesophageal dilator
5. Limiting the length of the wrap to 1.5 to 2.0 cm
6. Stabilizing the wrap to the esophagus by partial thickness bites of the esophagus during creation of the wrap

Although widely accepted, these key elements have not been tested in prospective randomized trials.

Early complications have mostly been minor and infrequent. Transient dysphagia occurs in nearly 50% and resolves within 3 weeks of surgery. An infrequent early problem, but one of greater concern, has been postoperative nausea and retching. During episodes of retching, breakdown of the fundoplication can occur. Therefore, postoperative nausea should be treated aggressively. Late complications of wrap migration and paraesophageal herniation may also be related to postoperative retching but more likely result from failure to close the esophageal hiatus or a shortened esophagus. Long-term dysphagia is emerging in 10% to 15% of patients but is well accepted by patients in the context of GERD symptom control. When a shortened esophagus is encountered, an esophageal lengthening procedure (Collis gastroplasty) may be used. However, esophageal lengthening is rarely indicated, and its use should be balanced with the findings that 80% of patients develop uncontrollable esophagitis or pathologic esophageal acid exposure.[22]

The Toupet fundoplication (**Fig. 3**) is identical to the Nissen except that the fundoplication is a 270° wrap rather than a 360° wrap. The gastric fundus is brought

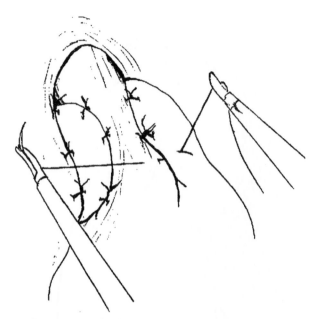

Fig. 3. Depiction of Toupet 270° fundoplication.

posterior to the esophagus and sutured to either side of the esophagus, leaving the anterior surface bare. This 270° fundoplication has the theoretic advantage of limiting postoperative bloating and dysphagia, especially in those with impaired esophageal body peristalsis. Many centers use the Toupet procedure exclusively in patients with abnormal esophageal peristalsis identified during preoperative esophageal manometry. Some have advocated the routine use of the Toupet fundoplication on all GERD patients, which could eliminate the need for preoperative esophageal manometry in many patients. However, it appears that a partial fundoplication is not as durable as a total fundoplication, and its use in the most severe cases (grade IV esophagitis, Barrett's esophagus, stricture) is questionable.[23]

Regardless of the technique used, the eight-fold increase in the use of ARS over the past decade has also exposed a larger cohort of patients in whom the procedure has failed. Failure rates range from 2% to 30% depending on the definition of failure. In select cases (eg, patients with symptomatic recurrent reflux) revisional fundoplication is offered, with most centers reporting a 3%–5% reoperation rate and a 65%–90% success rate. Wrap herniation is the leading cause of failure requiring reoperation, while wrap disruption, wrap slippage, too tight a fundoplication, and an undiagnosed motility disorder before the initial fundoplication are also frequently observed.[13]

CARE AFTER ARS

Patients are allowed to drink liquids immediately postoperatively. Carbonated beverages are specifically avoided due to the resulting gastric distension. Due to edema at the fundoplication, patients are maintained on a liquid diet for 5-7 days and then a soft diet for the next 2 weeks. Hospital dismissal is usually on the first postoperative day and follow-up in 3-4 weeks. In difficult cases (extensive paraesophageal dissection, redo surgery, or paraesophageal hernia repair), a contrast swallow on postoperative day one is recommended to rule out a small leak or other anatomic problems. Patients are released from the hospital with prescriptions for a liquid pain medicine, liquid stool softener, and an antiemetic that can be administered rectally should nausea occur. A dietician sees the patients before discharge to instruct them on the soft diet, emphasizing the avoidance of carbonated beverages, breads, and other dry foods that tend to lodge at the fundoplication. There are no limitations on physical activity unless there has been a paraesophageal hernia that has been repaired, in which case avoidance of heavy lifting is necessary for approximately 4–6 weeks. All preoperative antisecretory or prokinetic medications are stopped.

Postoperative nausea and vomiting/retching remain the most significant and controllable postoperative events associated with significant complications. Most patients receive preemptive antinausea medication, and staff caring for patients postoperatively are instructed to respond immediately with medication to any patient complaint of nausea. If any early postoperative retching occurs, a contrast swallow is immediately obtained in case wrap disruption or herniation has occurred. If this occurs and is detected within the first 24–48 hours, immediate reoperation can be undertaken to correct the problem. If these anatomic problems are not found until outpatient follow-up, a 6- to 12-week delay is necessary before undertaking reoperation due to the adhesions that will have formed by this time.

OUTCOMES OF ANTIREFLUX SURGERY

In the 1990s controlled trials that compared medical and surgical therapy of GERD favored surgical therapy.[9] Within these prospective randomized comparisons, surgical treatment was significantly more effective than medical therapy in improving symptoms and endoscopic signs of esophagitis for as long as 2 years. Other longitudinal studies report good to excellent long-term results in 80% to 93% of surgically treated patients.[24–28]

Thousands of patients undergoing laparoscopic Nissen fundoplication have been reported in the world's literature, with 93% of patients symptom free at 1 year postoperatively. Only 3% have required some medical therapy to control their symptoms. Overall, 97% of these patients are satisfied with their results. Transient dysphagia occurs in nearly 50% of patients and resolves within 3 weeks of surgery. Late complications of wrap migration and paraesophageal herniation may also be related to postoperative retching but are more likely due to failure to close the esophageal hiatus or a shortened esophagus. Long-term dysphagia is emerging in 10%–15% of patients, but it is frequently well accepted by patients in the context of the excellent GERD symptom control they experience. In 3%–4% of patients, unremitting dysphagia or recurrent reflux symptoms require reoperation for correction. When redo fundoplication is undertaken, 93% of patients experience good to excellent results. Troubling long-term side effects, such as gas bloat, have been virtually eliminated by the "floppy" nature of the fundoplication.

Although the goal of eliminating symptoms remains the primary concern, long-term follow-up of the controlled trials of the 1990s has raised questions regarding the durability of symptom control after ARS. In a follow-up to their original publication in 1992, Spechler and colleagues noted that 62% of the patients in the surgical treatment group participating in follow-up analysis took antireflux medications regularly. Additionally, they found no significant difference between the medical and surgical groups in the rate of esophagitis, esophageal strictures, esophageal cancer, or overall satisfaction.[29] Others have noted a similar number of patients requiring antisecretory medications more than 10 years following surgery.[27,30,31] Given a small, but not insignificant, mortality rate of 0.3% and the known associations with medium- to long-term postprandial bloating and diarrhea in up to 30%–45% of patients, this has led to a reappraisal of the role of ARS.[32] Ultimately, these data have helped patients become more informed about their choices in instituting a lifelong management plan.

To summarize, ARS is indicated in any patient with GERD refractory to medical management or who has symptom recurrence when medicine is withdrawn. In many patients with classic symptoms, an EGD and esophageal manometry are all the preoperative testing necessary. Additional tests are confirmatory in difficult cases. The laparoscopic Nissen fundoplication is both safe and effective in the long-term management of nearly all patients with chronic GERD. The Toupet fundoplication may be best used in patients with impaired esophageal body peristalsis.

ENDOSCOPIC ENDOLUMENAL THERAPY

Despite the advances made with the advent of laparoscopy, an ideal treatment for GERD that permanently alleviates symptoms, protects against esophageal erosion, and prevents malignant progression while minimizing the risk of therapy remains elusive. Recently, the search for this ideal therapy has led to the development of less invasive alternatives to medical and surgical therapy using endoscopy-based or endolumenal approaches. Now, patients who wish to avoid surgery searching for a nonpharmacologic solution can opt for procedures that require no skin incision and are often performed on an outpatient basis. The inherent allure of this approach has led several groups within industry to develop therapies designed to alter the anatomy or physiology of the gastroesophageal junction via the delivery of radiofrequency energy to the gastroesophageal junction, injection, or implantation of devices into the cardia and LES or suture plication of the proximal stomach.[33]

The clinical uses of radiofrequency energy have been well known for decades, ranging from the treatment of benign prostatic hyperplasia to hepatic tumor ablation. The delivery of radiofrequency energy to the esophagus and gastric cardia at a temperature of 65°C has been shown to cause collagen contraction and eventual tissue shrinkage, leading to scarring at the gastroesophageal junction and neurolysis in the same region. Although a clear understanding of the mechanism of action remains to be determined, it is thought that these anatomic changes induced by radiofrequency energy delivery decrease the frequency of transient LES relaxation episodes either via interference of afferent nerve signals to the brain or by decreasing the stimulation of gastric cardia mechanoreceptors through fibrosis or direct ablation.[34] The Stretta procedure characterizes this technique.

In 1984 O'Conner injected Teflon paste into the EG junction of 5 dogs with a surgically incompetent LES in an attempt to reverse GERD from within the distal esophagus. He noted that all reversed the preinjection levels of esophagitis with an improvement in reflux volume. Since that time, the concept of reversing GERD using an injectable substance at the LES has been actively investigated. Like radiofrequency ablation, no clear mechanism of action has been established. However, studies using an ethylene vinyl alcohol copolymer with tantalum dissolved in dimethyl sulfide (Enteryx, Boston Scientific Corporation, Natick, Massachusetts) injected into a porcine model led to an initial inflammatory reaction with eventual circumferential granulation and fibrous capsule formation (around the implant). It is hypothesized that this decreased the compliance of the distal esophagus and gastric cardia preventing shortening of the LES and possibly decreasing the number of transient lower esophageal relaxation episodes.[35] Placement of hydrogel implants into the submucosal space at the level of the LES (Gatekeeper, Medtronic, Minneapolis, Minnesota) increases the volume of the LES and is thought to create a barrier to gastric refluxate.[36]

The creation of intralumenal gastric pleats at the gastroesophageal junction is intended to mimic the effects of a gastric fundoplication by revising the anatomic alterations affecting the gastric cardia caused by chronic GERD. This is done via the deployment of staples or stitches through unique devices designed to work in tandem with standard esophagogastroscopes. Both partial- and full-thickness gastropexy techniques have been described under the trade names of EndoCinch (Bard), Plicator (NDO), and Esophyx (EndoGastric Solutions).[37–39] The physiologic impact of intralumenal gastroplication has been observed in both animals and humans, with an immediate increase in LES pressure, decrease in acid sensitivity, and decrease in the number of transient esophageal relaxation episodes detected.

Evidence regarding the effectiveness and safety of these procedures is still accumulating, primarily in the setting of proof-of-concept, small case study, cohort, or sham-comparison studies. Early results from cohort studies are promising, with therapies demonstrating improvements in quality of life (between 50% and 75% improvement), postprocedure symptom scores, PPI use (up to 40%–75%), 24-hour pH (16%–33% time, pH<4 improvement), and LES pressure. Randomized data reveal a trend in improvement of quality-of-life scores and medication use, with two studies noting improvements on objective evaluation (pH, EGD/esophagitis score/manometry). These findings suggest that endolumenal therapy may primarily play a role in the future in reducing symptoms and medication usage, with further evaluation required to fully understand the effects on the histopathological changes associated with GERD. Follow-up has been limited, thereby limiting conclusions as to the durability of the therapeutic effect. To date, report of one case control comparison of endoscopic suturing with laparoscopic Nissen fundoplication has been published.[40] Other sham-controlled trials have been completed on several of the techniques.[41–43]

As with any new therapy, questions of efficacy remain. Food and Drug Administration Phase III and IV data are only recently being evaluated. Perhaps more telling, and importantly, market forces are also influencing the availability of these therapies. Of the six companies offering some form of endolumenal therapy for GERD, four have either gone out of business or pulled the product from the market. Two companies remain, the first to enter this market (EndoCinch) and the last to enter this market (Esophyx). Until more data are accumulated, recommendations regarding the widespread use of endolumenal therapies for GERD outside of clinical trials cannot be made. The limitation that they are not suited to patients with hiatal herniation, Barrett's esophagus, or multiple comorbidities has been consistent across all of the proposed endolumenal therapies.

There is still promise that endolumenal therapies may serve as a means of symptom control, as a bridge to definitive therapy, as an alternative in mild to moderately symptomatic patients who do not desire surgery, as a more permanent therapeutic option for those who cannot tolerate surgical intervention, or as a less involved method of helping patients with recurrent reflux after ARS.

BARRETT'S ESOPHAGUS

Special mention is necessary for Barrett's esophagus. In 1950, Norman Barrett described the condition in which the tubular esophagus becomes lined with metaplastic columnar epithelium, which is at risk for adenocarcinoma. Most recently, it has been recognized that the specialized intestinal metaplasia (not gastric-type columnar changes) constitutes true Barrett's esophagus, with a risk of progression to dysplasia and adenocarcinoma.[44]

This abnormality occurs in 7% to 10% of people with GERD and may represent the end stage of the natural history of GERD. Clearly, Barrett's esophagus is associated with a more profound mechanical deficiency of the LES, severe impairment of esophageal body function, and marked esophageal acid exposure.[45] In contrast, some patients are asymptomatic and have only short segments of columnar lined epithelium in the distal esophagus (<3 cm), which does not have this same strong association with GERD. Additionally, there seems to be a lower incidence of metaplastic epithelium in these "short segments" of Barrett's and, therefore, a lower malignancy potential. There remains considerable debate regarding the significance of short-segment Barrett's esophagus, and identifying patients with so-called short-segment Barrett's esophagus remains problematic because endoscopically localizing the precise anatomic esophagogastric junction is difficult, and metaplastic epithelium (and, therefore, malignant potential) can exist even in these short segments. The endoscopic feature most strongly associated with intestinal metaplasia is the finding of long segments of esophageal columnar lining, with more than 90% of patients with greater than 3 cm of esophageal columnar lining having intestinal metaplasia.

Endoscopically obvious Barrett's esophagus with intestinal metaplasia is a major risk factor for adenocarcinoma of the esophagus, with the annual incidence of adenocarcinoma in this condition estimated at approximately 0.8%, 40 times higher than that in the general population. Once high-grade dysplasia is identified in more than one biopsy from columnar lined esophagus, nearly 50% of patients are found to already harbor foci of invasive cancer. This frequency is the basis for recommending careful endoscopic surveillance in patients with Barrett's esophagus with intestinal metaplasia and esophagectomy when high-grade dysplasia is identified.[46,47]

Treatment goals for patients with Barrett's esophagus are similar to those for patients with GERD, that is, relief of symptoms and arrest of ongoing reflux-mediated epithelial damage. Additionally, those with Barrett's esophagus, regardless of type of treatment (surgical or medical), require long-term endoscopic surveillance with biopsy of columnar segments to identify progressive metaplastic changes or progression to dysplasia.[48]

Several studies have compared medical and surgical therapy in patients with Barrett's esophagus. These data support the notion that Barrett's esophagus is associated with more severe and refractory GERD, and ARS is effective at alleviating these symptoms in 75% to 92% of patients. However, many patients are asymptomatic (perhaps explaining why they have such advanced sequelae of GERD), and there is mounting evidence to suggest that an alkaline refluxate may be as damaging as acid reflux.[49] For these reasons, correction of the mechanically defective antireflux barrier may be especially important in these patients.

Although symptom control in these patients suggests control of ongoing damage, the ultimate goal in therapy is to change the natural history in Barrett's esophagus of progression to adenocarcinoma. With this goal, several questions arise: (1) Does ARS result in regression of Barrett's epithelium?; (2) Does ARS prevent progression of metaplastic changes?; and (3) Is there a role for ARS accompanied by other therapies for metaplastic or dysplastic epithelium?

Does ARS result in regression of Barrett's epithelium? Operative therapy corrects the mechanically defective antireflux barrier, and, therefore, it might be expected to have a higher likelihood than medical therapy alone of inducing regression of Barrett's epithelium. In reviewing the results regarding regression with medical treatment, there is no substantial evidence that medical therapy results in regression. In a summary of several series, complete regression occurred in only six patients, with all but one coming from one series. Thirty-one patients showed some decrease in the length of Barrett's esophagus, but only six had a decrease in length of more than 1 cm. Furthermore, six patients went on to develop adenocarcinoma of the esophagus. In contrast, several studies now show regression with surgical therapy. In some series, up to 60% of patients have experienced visual regression and 40%, histologic.[50,51]

Does ARS prevent progression of metaplastic changes? There is growing evidence suggesting that ARS may prevent progression of Barrett's changes and thereby protect against dysplasia and malignancy. In a series reported by McDonald from the Mayo Clinic, three cancers occurred over an 18.5-year follow-up period, all within the first 3 years after operation.[52] The clustering of these three cases within the first 3 years of follow-up suggests that these patients may have already progressed to dysplasia at the time of operation. These are very strong data in support of the favorable impact of operative therapy on the natural history of Barrett's esophagus.

Is there a role for ARS accompanied by other therapies for metaplastic or dysplastic epithelium? Combination therapy, that is, pharmacologic or operative control of acid reflux plus endoscopic ablation of Barrett's mucosa, has encouraging preliminary results. These early experiences suggest that the ablated areas re-epithelialize with more normal squamous mucosa. Ablative therapies have included laser ablation, photodynamic therapy, and cryotherapy. A very promising newer therapy is radiofrequency ablation delivered via a tightly wound wire array around a balloon that can be inflated in the esophagus, thereby providing esophageal mucosal effacement with the delivery wires. When a short burst of high energy is delivered in this way, there appears to be uniform ablation of the esophageal mucosa without deep injury to the submucosa. With this, the ablation of the esophageal mucosa involved with Barrett's esophagus can be more uniform and predictable, and result in complete ablation with minimal risk of stricture or complications. Early studies using this technique are very promising.[53,54] This exciting early work needs further study before it becomes a clinical standard.

REFERENCES

1. Patti MG, Bresadola V. Gastroesophageal reflux disease: basic considerations. Problem in General Surgery 1996;13:1–8.
2. Wetscher GJ, Redmond EJ, Vititi LMH. Pathophysiology of gastroesophageal reflux disease. In: Hinder RA, editor. Gastroesophageal reflux disease. Austin: R.G. Landes Company; 1993. p. 7–29.
3. Dore MP, Pedroni A, Pes GM, et al. Effect of antisecretory therapy on atypical symptoms in gastroesophageal reflux disease. Dig Dis Sci 2007;52:463–8.
4. Long MD, Shaheen NJ. Extra-esophageal GERD: clinical dilemma of epidemiology versus clinical practice. Curr Gastroenterol Rep 2007;9:195–202.
5. Richter JE. The many manifestations of gastroesophageal reflux disease: presentation, evaluation, and treatment. Gastroenterol Clin North Am 2007;36:577–99.
6. Klingman RR, Stein HJ, DeMeester TR. The current management of gastroesophageal reflux. Adv Surg 1991;24:259–91.
7. Pace F, Tonini M, Pallotta S, et al. Systematic review: maintenance treatment of gastro-oesophageal reflux disease with proton pump inhibitors taken 'on-demand' [see comment]. Aliment Pharmacol Ther 2007;26:195–204.
8. Richter JE, Castell DO. Gastroesophageal reflux: pathogenesis, diagnosis and therapy. Ann Intern Med 1989;97:93–103.

9. Spechler SJ. Comparison of medical and surgical therapy for complicated gastroesophageal reflux disease in veterans. N Engl J Med 1992;326:786–92.

10. Laycock WS, Mauren S, Waring JP. Improvement in quality of life measures following laparoscopic antireflux surgery. Gastroenterology 1995;108:A244.

11. Sontag SJ. Gastroesophageal reflux and asthma. Am J Med 1997;103: 84S–90S.

12. Hunter JG, Smith CD, Branum GD, et al. Laparoscopic fundoplication failures: patterns of failure and response to fundoplication revision. Ann Surg 1999;230: 595–604.

13. Smith CD, McClusky DA, Rajad MA, et al. When fundoplication fails: redo? Ann Surg 2005;241:861–9.

14. Smith CD, Fink AS, Applegren K. Guidelines for surgical treatment of gastroesophageal reflux disease (GERD). Society of American Gastrointestinal Endoscopic Surgeons (SAGES). Surg Endosc 1998;12:186–8.

15. Eshraghi N, Farahmand M, Soot SJ, et al. Comparison of outcomes of open versus laparoscopic Nissen fundoplication performed in a single practice. Am J Surg 1998;175:371–4.

16. Anvari M, Allen C. Laparoscopic Nissen fundoplication: two-year comprehensive follow-up of a technique of minimal paraesophageal dissection. Ann Surg 1998; 227:25–32.

17. Anvari M, Allen C, Borm A. Laparoscopic Nissen fundoplication is a satisfactory alternative to long-term omeprazole therapy. Br J Surg 1995;82:938–42.

18. Bloomston M, Zervos E, Gonzalez R, et al. Quality of life and antireflux medication use following laparoscopic Nissen fundoplication. Am Surg 1998;64:509–13.

19. Champault G, Volter F, Rizk N, et al. Gastroesophageal reflux: conventional surgical treatment versus laparoscopy. A prospective study of 61 cases. Surg Laparosc Endosc 1996;6:434–40.

20. Hinder RA, Filipi CJ, Wetscher G, et al. Laparoscopic Nissen fundoplication is an effective treatment for gastroesophageal reflux disease. Ann Surg 1994;220: 472–81.

21. Hunter JG, Trus TL, Branum DG, et al. A physiologic approach to laparoscopic fundoplication for gastroesophageal reflux disease. Ann Surg 1996; 223:673–87.

22. Lin E, Swafford V, Chadalavada R, et al. Disparity between symptomatic and physiologic outcomes following esophageal lengthening procedures for antireflux surgery. J Gastrointest Surg 2004;8:31–9.

23. Farrell TM, Smith CD, Archer SB, et al. Heartburn is more likely to recur after Toupet fundoplication than Nissen fundoplication. American Surgeon 2000;66: 229–37.

24. Macintyre IM, Goulbourne IA. Long-term results after Nissen fundoplication: a 5-15-year review. J R Coll Surg Edinb 1990;35:159–62.

25. Mark LA, Okrainec A, Ferri LE, et al. Comparison of patient-centered outcomes after laparoscopic Nissen fundoplication for gastroesophageal reflux disease or paraesophageal hernia. Surg Endosc 2008;22:343–7.

26. Morgenthal CB, Lin E, Shane MD, et al. Who will fail laparoscopic Nissen fundoplication? Preoperative prediction of long-term outcomes. Surg Endosc 2007;21: 1978–84.

27. Morgenthal CB, Shane MD, Stival A, et al. The durability of laparoscopic Nissen fundoplication: 11-year outcomes. J Gastrointest Surg 2007;11:693–700.

28. Pope CE II. The quality of life following antireflux surgery. World J Surg 1992;16: 355–8.

29. Spechler SJ, Lee E, Ahnen D, et al. Long-term outcome of medical and surgical therapies for gastroesophageal reflux disease: follow-up of a randomized controlled trial [see comment]. JAMA 2001;285:2331–8.

30. Liu JY, Woloshin S, Laycock WS, et al. Late outcomes after laparoscopic surgery for gastroesophageal reflux. Arch Surg 2002;137:397–401.

31. Zaninotto G, Portale G, Costantini M, et al. Long-term results (6–10 years) of laparoscopic fundoplication. J Gastrointest Surg 2007;11:1138–45.

32. Richter JE. Let the patient beware: the evolving truth about laparoscopic antireflux surgery. [comment]. Am J Med 2003;114:71–3.

33. Falk GW, Fennerty MB, Rothstein RI. AGA Institute technical review on the use of endoscopic therapy for gastroesophageal reflux disease. Gastroenterology 2006;131:1315–36.

34. Utley DS, Kim M, Vierra MA, et al. Augmentation of lower esophageal sphincter pressure and gastric yield pressure after radiofrequency energy delivery to the gastroesophageal junction: a porcine model. Gastrointest Endosc 2000;52:81–6.

35. Mason RJ, Hughes M, Lehman GA, et al. Endoscopic augmentation of the cardia with a biocompatible injectable polymer (Enteryx) in a porcine model [see comment]. Surg Endosc 2002;16:386–91.

36. Fockens P, Bruno MJ, Gabbrielli A, et al. Endoscopic augmentation of the lower esophageal sphincter for the treatment of gastroesophageal reflux disease: multicenter study of the Gatekeeper Reflux Repair System. Endoscopy 2004;36:682–9.

37. Cadiere GB, Rajan A, Rqibate M, et al. Endoluminal fundoplication (ELF)–evolution of EsophyX, a new surgical device for transoral surgery. Minim Invasive Ther Allied Technol 2006;15:348–55.

38. Mahmood Z, McMahon BP, Arfin Q, et al. Endocinch therapy for gastrooesophageal reflux disease: a one year prospective follow up [see comment]. Gut 2003;52:34–9.

39. Tam WC, Holloway RH, Dent J, et al. Impact of endoscopic suturing of the gastroesophageal junction on lower esophageal sphincter function and gastroesophageal reflux in patients with reflux disease [see comment]. Am J Gastroenterol 2004;99:195–202.

40. Chadalavada R, Lin E, Swafford V, et al. Comparative results of endoluminal gastroplasty and laparoscopic antireflux surgery for the treatment of GERD. Surg Endosc 2004;18:261–5.

41. Corley DA, Katz P, Wo JM, et al. Improvement of gastroesophageal reflux symptoms after radiofrequency energy: a randomized, sham-controlled trial [see comment]. Gastroenterology 2003;125:668–76.

42. Deviere J, Costamagna G, Neuhaus H, et al. Nonresorbable copolymer implantation for gastroesophageal reflux disease: a randomized sham-controlled multicenter trial [see comment]. Gastroenterology 2005;128:532–40.

43. Montgomery M, Hakanson B, Ljungqvist O, et al. Twelve months' follow-up after treatment with the EndoCinch endoscopic technique for gastrooesophageal reflux disease: a randomized, placebo-controlled study. Scand J Gastroenterol 2006;41:1382–9.

44. Van Blankenstein M, Looman CW, Kruijshaar ME, et al. Modelling a population with Barrett's oesophagus from oesophageal adenocarcinoma incidence data. Scand J Gastroenterol 2007;42:308–17.

45. Peters JH. The surgical management of Barrett's esophagus. Gastroenterol Clin North Am 1997;26:647–68.

46. Edwards MJ, Gable DR, Lentsch AB, et al. The rationale for esophagectomy as the optimal therapy for Barrett's esophagus with high-grade dysplasia. Ann Surg 1996;223:585–9.
47. Heitmiller RF, Redmond M, Hamilton SR. Barrett's esophagus with high-grade dysplasia. An indication for prophylactic esophagectomy. Ann Surg 1996;224: 66–71.
48. Society for Surgery of the Alimentary T. SSAT patient care guidelines. Management of Barrett's esophagus. J Gastrointest Surg 2007;11:1213–5.
49. Dixon MF, Neville PM, Mapstone NP, et al. Bile reflux gastritis and Barrett's oesophagus: further evidence of a role for duodenogastro-oesophageal reflux? Gut 2001;49:359–63.
50. Rossi M, Barreca M, de Bortoli N, et al. Efficacy of Nissen fundoplication versus medical therapy in the regression of low-grade dysplasia in patients with Barrett esophagus: a prospective study [see comment]. Ann Surg 2006;243:58–63.
51. Sharma P. Barrett esophagus: will effective treatment prevent the risk of progression to esophageal adenocarcinoma? Am J Med 2004;117(Suppl 5A):79S–85S.
52. McDonald ML, Trastek VF, Allen MS, et al. Barrett's esophagus: does an antireflux procedure reduce the need for endoscopic surveillance? J Thorac Cardiovasc Surg 1996;111:1135–8.
53. Dunkin BJ, Martinez J, Bejarano PA, et al. Thin-layer ablation of human esophageal epithelium using a bipolar radiofrequency balloon device. Surg Endosc 2006;20:125–30.
54. Smith CD, Bejarano PA, Melvin WS, et al. Endoscopic ablation of intestinal metaplasia containing high-grade dysplasia in esophagectomy patients using a balloon-based ablation system. Surg Endosc 2007;21:560–9.

Assessment of Gastric Emptying and Small-Bowel Motility: Scintigraphy, Breath Tests, Manometry, and SmartPill

Henry P. Parkman, MD

KEYWORDS

- Gastric emptying • Gastric emptying breath tests
- Antroduodenal manometry • Capsule motility

Gastrointestinal (GI) motility and functional GI disorders are common reasons for patients to see gastroenterologists. Patients with symptoms suggesting these disorders are commonly encountered by a variety of physicians, especially gastroenterologists. In most patients, the physical examination and upper endoscopy are normal, and thus symptoms are suggested to be from a motility disorder or a functional GI disorder. Knowledge of the evaluation and treatment of these disorders is important to appropriately care for these patients in clinical practice.

Gastric dysmotility is important in several clinical disorders, including gastroparesis and functional dyspepsia. Symptoms of gastroparesis may overlap with those of functional dyspepsia. Delayed gastric emptying (GE), impaired gastric accommodation to a meal, and visceral hypersensitivity are 3 potential pathophysiologic factors in functional dyspepsia. Interestingly, some patients with functional dyspepsia may have rapid GE. Proper evaluation to help distinguish the pathophysiologic basis of the patient's symptoms might help direct proper medical treatment.

Regional properties of the stomach are important for normal processing of ingested food. The main functions of gastric motility are accommodation with relaxation of the proximal stomach to serve as a reservoir for ingested food, trituration in the distal stomach to grind down solid particles, and controlled emptying of chyme into the duodenum. GE reflects integration of the propulsive forces of the proximal gastric (fundic) tone and distal gastric (antral) contractions with inhibitory forces of the pylorus. Gastric dysmotility includes altered GE, antral hypomotility, impaired fundic

Temple University School of Medicine, Gastroenterology Section, Parkinson Pavilion, 8th Floor, 3401 North Broad Street, Philadelphia, PA 19140, USA
E-mail address: henry.parkman@temple.edu

Gastrointest Endoscopy Clin N Am 19 (2009) 49–55
doi:10.1016/j.giec.2008.12.003
1052-5157/08/$ – see front matter © 2009 Elsevier Inc. All rights reserved.

accommodation, pyloric sphincter dysfunction, and gastric dysrhythmias. Appropriate testing can evaluate each of these physiologic processes of gastric motility. Tests of gastric motility include evaluation of GE, recording contractile pressures, recording gastric myoelectric activity, measuring gastric accommodation, and more recently, satiety testing, which tests accommodation and sensitivity.

Small-bowel dysmotility can include disorders from small-intestinal pseudo-obstruction to irritable bowel syndrome. The disorders can be neurogenic or myogenic in origin. Small-bowel dysmotility can give rise to bacterial overgrowth, which can also cause symptoms including bloating and diarrhea.

GASTROPARESIS

Gastroparesis is a disorder characterized by symptoms of and evidence for gastric retention in the absence of mechanical obstruction. Gastroparesis typically affects patients, mostly women, and has significant impact on quality of life. The true prevalence of gastroparesis is not known; however, it has been estimated that up to 4% of the population experiences symptomatic manifestations of this condition. Diabetes mellitus is the most common systemic disease associated with gastroparesis. A similar number of patients present with gastroparesis of an idiopathic nature. Postsurgical gastroparesis, often with vagotomy or damage to the vagus nerve, represents the third most common etiology of gastroparesis. The most frequently reported symptoms of gastroparesis include nausea, vomiting, early satiety, and postprandial fullness. Abdominal discomfort and pain are also noted by many affected patients and represent challenging symptoms to treat. Weight loss, malnutrition, and dehydration may be prominent in severe cases. In diabetics, gastroparesis may adversely affect glycemic control.

Although it has been a common assumption that the GI symptoms can be attributed to delay in GE, most investigations have observed only weak correlations between symptom severity and the degree of gastric stasis. Early studies suggested that symptom severity in gastroparesis does not correlate well with the degree of gastric stasis. Recent studies report that early satiety, postprandial fullness, and vomiting correlate with delayed emptying in functional dyspepsia. A symptom questionnaire, the Gastroparesis Cardinal Symptom Index (GCSI), has been developed and validated in university-based clinical practices for quantifying symptoms in gastroparesis. The GCSI is based on three subscales (postprandial fullness/early satiety, nausea/vomiting, and bloating) and represents a subset of the longer Patient Assessment of Upper Gastrointestinal Disorders-Symptoms.

The diagnosis of gastroparesis is made when a delay in GE is present and laboratory studies rule out metabolic causes of symptoms and endoscopic and/or radiographic testing excludes luminal blockage. The classic test for measurement of GE is scintigraphy using an egg meal cooked with a technetium radiolabel with imaging out to 4 hours postprandially. Two new methods are available to measure GE. First, a pH and pressure recording capsule, SmartPill (SmartPill Corporation; www.smartpillcorp.com), which was approved by the Food and Drug Administration (FDA) in 2007, can assess GE by the acidic gastric residence time of the capsule as measured by the duration of acidity from capsule ingestion to the change in pH from the acidic stomach to the alkaline duodenum. This capsule can also record pressures throughout the GI tract. Secondly, a ^{13}C-octanoate breath test (OBT) can be used for measuring GE and has been shown to correlate significantly with GE for solids by scintigraphy. A muffin-based OBT is convenient, sensitive, and specific to detect delayed GE. These tests are discussed in depth below.

GE SCINTIGRAPHY

GE scintigraphy (GES) of a solid-phase meal is considered the gold standard for the diagnosis of gastroparesis because this test quantifies the emptying of a physiologic caloric meal. In patients with gastroparesis, liquid emptying may remain normal until the disorder is at an advanced stage. Liquid-phase emptying scans are more commonly performed after gastric surgery in patients suspected of having dumping syndrome. The usefulness of gastric scintigraphy in directing therapy and predicting response has been debated.

For solid-phase testing, most centers use a ^{99m}Tc sulfur colloid–labeled egg sandwich as a test meal. In 2008, a meal using Egg Beaters egg whites with standard imaging at 0, 1, 2, and 4 hours postprandially has been proposed to provide a degree of standardization between different centers. Scintigraphic assessment of emptying should be extended to at least 2 hours and preferably 4 hours after meal ingestion. A recent consensus statement from members of the American Neurogastroenterology and Motility Society and the Society of Nuclear Medicine recommended this standardized method for measuring GES. The low-fat egg white meal with imaging at 0, 1, 2, and 4 hours after meal ingestion, as described by a published multicenter protocol by Tougas and colleagues, provides standardized information about normal and delayed GE. Adoption of this standardized protocol will resolve the lack of uniformity of testing, add reliability and credibility to the results, and improve the clinical utility of the GE test. Even with extension of the scintigraphic study to this length, there may be significant day-to-day variability (up to 20%) in rates of GE. For shorter durations, the test is less reliable due to larger variations of normal GE. Extending scintigraphy to 4 hours has been advocated by several investigators to improve the accuracy in determining the presence of gastroparesis.

Emptying of solids typically exhibits a lag phase followed by a prolonged linear emptying phase. A variety of parameters can be calculated from the emptying profile of a radiolabeled meal. The simplest approach for interpreting a GE study is to report the percent retention at defined times after meal ingestion (usually 2 and 4 hours). The half-emptying time may also be calculated; however, extrapolation of the emptying curve from an individual who did not empty 50% of the ingested meal during the actual imaging time may provide an inaccurate determination of the half-emptying time.

Patients should discontinue medications that may affect GE for an adequate period before this test based on drug half-life. For most medications, this will be 48 to 72 hours. Opiate analgesics and anticholinergic agents delay GE. Prokinetic agents that accelerate emptying may give a falsely normal GE result. Serotonin receptor antagonists such as ondansetron, which have little effect on GE, may be given for severe symptoms before performance of gastric scintigraphy. Hyperglycemia (glucose level >270 mg/dL) delays GE in diabetic patients. It is not unreasonable to defer GE testing until relative euglycemia is achieved to obtain a reliable determination of emptying parameters in the absence of acute metabolic derangement. Premenopausal women have slower GE than men; some centers primarily in Europe use separate reference values for premenopausal women.

Dual labeling of solids with ^{99m}Tc and liquids with ^{111}In allows for assessment of GE of solids and liquids, which may be useful for patients after gastric surgery to assess their differential handling by the postsurgical stomach and for patients who have undergone gastric surgery to determine whether symptoms might result from delayed solid emptying or rapid liquid emptying. Continued imaging of ^{111}In may be used to assess small-bowel transit, which is measured by the percent activity reaching the terminal ileum/cecum/ascending colon region of interest. Further imaging over the next several days provides an assessment of colonic transit, which can be quantitated using a geometric center of the radioactivity.

GE measures only the net output of solids or liquids from the stomach and fails to define the pathophysiologic mechanisms that may contribute to impair GE. Recent technical advances in scintigraphy provide information on fundic and antral abnormalities. Regional GE can assess intragastric meal distribution and transit from the proximal to distal portions of the stomach. Proximal retention has been described in gastroesophageal reflux disease, distal retention in functional dyspepsia, and global retention in gastroparesis. Dynamic antral contraction scintigraphy with frequent imaging can visualize antral contractions.

BREATH TESTING FOR GE

Breath tests using the nonradioactive isotope ^{13}C bound to a digestible substance have been validated for measuring GE. Most commonly, ^{13}C-labeled octanoate, a medium-chain triglyceride, is bound into a solid meal such as a muffin. Other studies have bound ^{13}C to acetate or to proteinaceous algae (*Spirulina*). After ingestion and stomach emptying, ^{13}C-octanoate is absorbed in the small intestine and metabolized to $^{13}CO_2$, which is then expelled from the lungs during respiration. The rate-limiting step is the rate of solid GE. Thus, octanoate breath testing provides a measure of solid-phase emptying. The octanoate breath test provides reproducible results that correlate with findings on GES. ^{13}C breath tests do not use ionizing radiation and can be used to test patients in the community or even at the bedside, where gamma camera facilities are not readily available. Breath samples can be preserved and shipped to a laboratory for analysis. Most octanoate breath testing is performed for clinical research and pharmaceutical studies. The penetrance of this diagnostic modality into clinical practice has been limited, although recent studies suggest that this test might be comparable to GES. Validation of this test in patients with emphysema, cirrhosis, celiac sprue, and pancreatic insufficiency is needed, because rates of octanoate metabolism may be impaired in these disorders.

pH AND PRESSURE SENSING CAPSULE (SMARTPILL)

The SmartPill is an ingestible capsule that measures pH, pressure, and temperature using miniaturized wireless sensor technology. The SmartPill capsule is swallowed by the patient and information is recorded as to acidity and pressures as it travels through the entire GI tract. From these measurements, GE and total GI tract transit time can be obtained. In addition, the SmartPill capsule will characterize pressure patterns and provide motility indices for the stomach, small intestine, and colon. Thus, SmartPill capsule aids in evaluation of patients with symptoms of GI motility disorders and functional GI disorders, such as gastroparesis.

The SmartPill is aimed at evaluating patients with possible GI motility and functional GI disorders. Studies have shown that the SmartPill provides information on GE and total GI transit time. It is useful to evaluate patients suspected to have gastroparesis. Gastroparesis, or slow GE, is a condition that affects a wide range of patients, including up to an estimated 40% of diabetics and those suffering from Parkinson disease. Studies suggest that the SmartPill is useful in assessing colonic transit and whole gut transit in patients with constipation with similar results to those in radiopaque markers.

The SmartPill GI Monitoring System was recently approved by the FDA for the assessment of gastric pH, GE, and total GI transit time. The SmartPill GI Monitoring System is indicated for use in evaluating patients with suspected delayed GE (gastroparesis). Delayed GE is implicated in such disorders as idiopathic and diabetic gastroparesis and functional nonulcer dyspepsia.

The SmartPill's physiologic measurements are used to determine GE time, total transit time, and combined small- and large-bowel transit time. In addition, pressure contraction patterns from the antrum and duodenum are used to calculate motility indices.

ELECTROGASTROGRAPHY

Electrogastrography (EGG) records gastric myoelectrical activity, known as the slow wave, using cutaneous electrodes affixed to the anterior abdomen overlying the stomach. The slow wave is responsible for controlling the maximal frequency and the controlled aboral propagation of distal gastric contractions. The normal gastric slow-wave frequency is approximately 3 cpm. Meal ingestion increases the amplitude of the EGG signal, which is believed to result either from increased antral contractility or from mechanical distention of the stomach. EGG testing quantifies the dominant frequency and regularity of gastric myoelectrical activity and the percentage of time in which abnormal slow-wave rhythms are present during fasting and postprandially; and it assesses the increase in amplitude (or power) after a meal. In general, an abnormal EGG result is defined when the percentage of time in dysrhythmias exceeds 30% of the recording time and/or when meal ingestion fails to elicit an increase in signal amplitude.

Gastric dysrhythmias (tachygastria, bradygastria) and decreased EGG amplitude responses to meal ingestion have been characterized in patients with idiopathic and diabetic gastroparesis. Gastric myoelectric abnormalities have also been described in patients with unexplained nausea and vomiting, motion sickness, and nausea and vomiting of pregnancy. EGG abnormalities are present in 75% of patients with gastro-paresis versus 25% of symptomatic patients with normal GE. Some investigators suggest that EGG abnormalities and delayed GE may define slightly different patient populations with dyspeptic symptoms. Symptomatic responses to antiemetic or pro-kinetic drug treatments have correlated better with resolution of gastric dysrhythmias than acceleration of delayed emptying in some patient subsets. Hyperglycemia may provoke dysrhythmias in diabetic patients.

Clinically, EGG has been used to demonstrate gastric myoelectric abnormalities in patients with unexplained nausea and vomiting or functional dyspepsia. EGG is considered an adjunct to GES as part of a comprehensive evaluation of patients with refractory symptoms suggestive of an upper GI motility disorder. However, to date, there has been little investigation to validate the utility of EGG in the management of patients with suspected gastric dysmotility.

ANTRODUODENAL MANOMETRY

Antroduodenojejunal (small-bowel) manometry (ADM) provides information about coordination of gastric and small-intestinal motor function in both fasting and post-prandial periods. Small-bowel manometry helps to identify normal motility features and consequently to identify abnormal motor patterns. The procedure is somewhat invasive and lengthy (requiring at least 5 hours of recording) and performed at only select centers. Ambulatory studies can also be performed over 24 hours using solid-state transducers and allow for correlation of symptoms with abnormal motility. However, catheter migration in the stomach during the ambulatory study prevents quantitation of antral contractility. Medications may affect small-intestinal motility—both transit and contractility. Most of these medications should be stopped 2 days before tests of small-intestinal manometry.

Patients who remain undiagnosed after extensive traditional workup and fail several courses of medical therapy should be referred for small-bowel manometry. The main indications for ADM are to evaluate (1) unexplained nausea and vomiting; (2) the cause of gastric or small-bowel stasis (eg, differentiation of neuropathic or myopathic disorders); and (3) suspected chronic intestinal pseudo-obstruction when the diagnosis is unclear.

ADM may differentiate between a neuropathic or myopathic motility disorder and may suggest unexpected small-bowel obstruction or rumination syndrome. Myopathic disorders, such as scleroderma, amyloidosis, or hollow visceral myopathy, have low-amplitude (<20 mm Hg) contractions with normal propagation. Neuropathic disorders have normal amplitude but abnormal propagative contractions, seen readily in phase III migratory motor complex (MMC), such as bursts and sustained uncoordinated pressure activity, and a failure of a meal to induce the fed type pattern. Occult mechanical obstruction of the small intestine is suggested by nonpropagated, prolonged contractions during the postprandial period. ADM may demonstrate a characteristic pattern of rumination with an increase in intra-abdominal pressures that occurs at all levels of the upper gut (R waves), especially postprandially. Clustered contractions may suggest irritable bowel syndrome, although these can be seen in other conditions.

Antral contractility is also measured during ADM. Decreased antral contractility and phase III MMCs originating in the small intestine rather than in the stomach can be seen in gastroparesis. ADM can help confirm or exclude a gastric motility disorder if the GE test is normal or borderline. With an accurate stationary recording, a reduced postprandial distal antral motility index is correlated with impaired GE of solids. A normal study with a normal transit test strongly suggests that motor dysfunction is not the cause of symptoms.

Some investigators perform the study with administration of erythromycin and/or octreotide to predict the patient's response to chronic treatment of these agents. In pediatric studies, the absence of MMCs is an indicator of a poor response to prokinetic agents.

Satiety Testing

Satiety testing with symptom-limited consumption of a test liquid has been proposed as a noninvasive technique to evaluate accommodation. In the water load test, the patient drinks water until he or she feels very full. Other investigators have used nutrient-containing test meals that are consumed at a fixed slow rate until satiety is achieved. Results of satiety testing correlate with the degree of gastric accommodation as measured by a barostat. Satiety tests offer the potential to noninvasively evaluate for abnormalities of gastric accommodation and perhaps visceral sensitivity. To date, most studies have quantified defects in satiety in patients with functional dyspepsia. Low volumes are consumed in patients with functional dyspepsia compared with those in normal controls. The test is becoming increasingly used in pharmacologic research studies. Investigations characterizing responses to satiety testing have not been reported in patients with gastroparesis.

SUMMARY

This article has reviewed tests to evaluate patients with upper GI symptoms suggesting disordered motility of the stomach and small intestine. Several tests are available for the evaluation of patients with suspected gastroparesis, including scintigraphy and the SmartPill. Breath testing for GE may be available in the near future. Proper evaluation of the stomach and small-bowel motility may help one to arrive at a correct diagnosis for patients with unexplained upper GI symptoms and may help enable proper treatment of the patient.

FURTHER READINGS

Abell TL, Camilleri M, Donohoe K, et al. Consensus recommendations for gastric emptying scintigraphy. A joint report of the Society of Nuclear Medicine and The American Neurogastroenterology and Motility Society. Am J Gastroenterol 2008;103:753–63.

Bouras EP, Delgado-Aros S, Camilleri M, et al. SPECT imaging of the stomach: comparison with barostat, and effects of sex, age, body mass index, and fundoplication. Single photon emission computed tomography. Gut 2002;51(6):781–6.

Bromer MQ, Kantor SN, Wagner DA, et al. Simultaneous measurement of gastric emptying with a simple muffin meal using 13C-octanoate breath test and scintigraphy in normal subjects and patients with dyspeptic symptoms. Dig Dis Sci 2002;47:1657–63.

Camilleri M, Hasler W, Parkman HP, et al. Measurement of gastroduodenal motility in the GI laboratory. Gastroenterology 1998;115:747–62.

Guo J-P, Maurer AH, Urbain J-L, et al. Extending gastric emptying scintigraphy from two to four hours detects more patients with gastroparesis. Dig Dis Sci 2001;46: 24–9.

Knight LC, Parkman HP, Brown KL, et al. Delayed gastric emptying and decreased antral contractility in normal premenopausal women compared to men. Am J Gastroenterol 1997;92:968–75.

Kuo B, McCallum RW, Koch K, et al. Comparison of gastric emptying of a non-digestible capsule to a radiolabeled meal in healthy and gastroparetic subjects. Aliment Pharmacol Ther 2008;27(2):186–96.

Parkman HP, Hasler WL, Barnett JL, et al. Electrogastrography: a document prepared by the gastric section of the American motility society clinical GI motility testing task force. Neurogastroenterol Motil 2003;15:488–97.

Parkman HP, Hasler WL, Fisher RS. American Gastroenterological Association technical review on diagnosis and treatment of gastroparesis. Gastroenterology 2004;127:1592–622.

Quigley EMM, Hasler WL, Parkman HP. AGA technical review on nausea and vomiting. Gastroenterology 2001;120:263–86.

Stanghellini V, Tosetti C, Paternico A, et al. Risk indicators of delayed gastric emptying of solids in patients with functional dyspepsia. Gastroenterology 1996;110: 1036–42.

Simonian HP, Kantor S, Knight LC, et al. Simultaneous assessment of gastric accommodation and emptying: Studies with liquid and solid meals. J Nucl Med 2004;45: 1155–60.

Tougas G, Eaker EY, Abell TL, et al. Assessment of gastric emptying using a low fat meal: establishment of international control values. Am J Gastroenterol 2000;95: 1456–62.

Current Treatment of Nausea and Vomiting Associated with Gastroparesis: Antiemetics, Prokinetics, Tricyclics

Jeremy Stapleton, DO, John M. Wo, MD*

KEYWORDS

- Gastroparesis • Nausea • Vomiting • Antiemetics
- Prokinetics • Tricyclics

Gastroparesis is a symptomatic chronic syndrome characterized by delayed gastric emptying without a mechanical obstruction.[1,2] It is the most common true motility disorder of the stomach. Delayed gastric emptying can be found in 40% to 65% of unselected diabetic individuals,[3,4] but only 6% to 17% of diabetics in the community report nausea or vomiting.[5,6] To establish a diagnosis of gastroparesis, delayed gastric emptying should be contributing to the patient's symptoms. However, the cause and effect relationship between delayed gastric emptying and symptom generation can be difficult to prove.

Any disease state that affects the gastrointestinal smooth muscle, autonomic nervous system, or enteric nervous system can cause or contribute to gastroparesis.[2] The potential causes of gastroparesis are numerous (**Table 1**). The most common established causes of gastroparesis are diabetes and postsurgical complications. Postsurgical gastroparesis can result from procedures with or without vagotomy. Central and peripheral autonomic disorders can involve the vagus nerve, resulting in gastroparesis. Connective tissue disorders such as scleroderma can cause abnormalities of motility in different regions of the gastrointestinal tract, potentially leading to gastroparesis, secondary aperistalsis, or chronic intestinal pseudo-obstruction. Paraneoplastic syndromes in which the cancer cells express antigens that mimic the neuronal tissues can result in an inflammatory neuropathy of the enteric nervous

Division of Gastroenterology/Hepatology, Department of Medicine, University of Louisville School of Medicine, 550 S Jackson Street, ACB 3rd floor, Louisville, KY 40202, USA
* Corresponding author.
E-mail address: johnwo@louisville.edu (J.M. Wo).

Gastrointest Endoscopy Clin N Am 19 (2009) 57–72
doi:10.1016/j.giec.2008.12.008
1052-5157/08/$ – see front matter © 2009 Elsevier Inc. All rights reserved.

Table 1	
Potential Causes of Gastroparesis	
Endocrine diseases	Diabetes
	Hypothyroidism
	Renal failure
Postsurgical	Procedures with vagotomy
	Partial or complete gastrectomy
	Esophagectomy
	Procedures without vagotomy
	Fundoplication
	Bariatric surgery
	Heart–lung transplant
Neuromuscular diseases	Multiple sclerosis
	Chronic idiopathic demyelinating
	polyneuropathy
	Myotonic dystrophy
Connective tissue diseases	Scleroderma
	Mixed connective tissue disorder
	Polymyositis
	Dermatomyositis
Autonomic diseases	Central
	Parkinson disease
	Multiple system atrophy
	Lewy body disease
	Brainstem diseases
	Peripheral
	Idiopathic dysautonomia
	Amyloidosis
	Vitamin B12 deficiency
	Mitochondrial disorder
	Porphyria
Paraneoplastic syndrome	Small cell lung cancer
	Multiple myeloma
	Breast cancer
	Lymphomas
Medications	Opiates
	Anticholinergics
	TCAs
	Calcium channel blockers
	Dopamine agonists for Parkinson disease
	and restless legs syndrome
Infection	Virus
	Epstein-Barr
	Cytomegalovirus
	Herpes simplex
	Norwalk virus
	Rotavirus
	Parasites
	Trypanosoma cruzi (Chagas disease)

system. However, the underlying cause of gastroparesis may not be found in about 40% of patients, a condition called idiopathic gastroparesis.[7]

Gastroparesis is frequently overlooked in clinical practice, because the symptoms are nonspecific. Some patients may present with regurgitation-predominant symptoms suggestive of gastroesophageal reflux disease, but effortless regurgitation of undigested foods should suggest gastroparesis.[8] Others may have prominent postprandial distress suggestive of functional dyspepsia. The most recognized symptoms of gastroparesis are chronic or episodic nausea, retching, and vomiting, which may result in dehydration, weight loss, and hospitalization. The number of gastroparesis-related hospitalizations is increasing in the United States, suggesting that the prevalence of gastroparesis is also increasing.[9] Gastroparesis, especially idiopathic gastroparesis, is a very heterogeneous syndrome with multiple factors contributing to symptoms. The cause and effect relationship between symptom generation and delayed gastric emptying is often difficult to prove. Multiple pharmacologic interventions are often needed in the treatment of gastroparesis. This review provides an update on the use of antiemetics, prokinetics, and tricyclics for the treatment of nausea and vomiting associated with gastroparesis.

MECHANISMS OF NAUSEA AND VOMITING

Nausea is a subjective sensation and is difficult to define.[10] Patients often feel they are about to vomit, or they use terms such as "sick to the stomach" or "queasy." Nausea is also difficult to measure. Different dimensions of nausea, such as maximal intensity, entity, duration, and quantity, should be incorporated in assessing the severity of nausea.[11] In contrast, vomiting is a specific event that results in retching and forceful evacuation of gastric contents in retrograde fashion from the stomach up to and out of the mouth.[10]

The pathophysiology of nausea and vomiting is complex. Induction of nausea and vomiting may originate from internal signals within our body or from external stimuli from our environment. Signals from the pharynx, stomach, and small intestine are transmitted via the parasympathetic and sympathetic visceral afferent pathways to the nucleus tractus solitarius in the medulla. This is likely the most common pathophysiology associated with gastroparesis, where gastric distension or other signals stimulate visceral afferent input to the central nervous system (CNS) resulting in vomiting. Integrity of the abdominal vagus is essential for the act of emesis.[12] Retching and vomiting may be absent if these pathways are not activated, such as in patients with postvagotomy gastroparesis with effortless regurgitation of undigested foods or in patients with dyspepsia-predominant gastroparesis.[8] However, the precise pathophysiology of nausea and vomiting associated with gastroparesis has yet to be identified.

The chemoreceptor trigger zone, which is located in the area postrema on the floor of the fourth ventricle, lies outside the blood–brain barrier and detects endogenous and exogenous toxins that induce emesis. Contrary to the common belief, there is no isolated "vomiting center" that causes emesis; rather it is a group of loosely organized neurons in the medulla that receive signals from the nucleus tractus solitarius and the chemoreceptor trigger zone.[12] There is an abundance of 5-hydroxytryptamine 3 (5-HT3) receptors in the chemoreceptor trigger zone. Vagal and sympathetic input stimulates the 5-HT3 receptors, leading to the release of dopamine. This dopamine surge activates the dopamine-2 receptors in the medulla. This complex pathway is the basis for the antiemetic properties of the pharmacologic agents that block the 5-HT3 and dopamine-2 receptors.

Nausea and vomiting may also arise from the vestibular system pathway, which contains numerous histamine-1 and muscarinic-1 receptors. The vestibular center is the prominent mechanism in motion sickness and pregnancy-induced nausea and vomiting, but it plays a less prominent pathophysiologic role in gastroparesis.

However, histamine-1 and muscarinic-1 receptor antagonists may be useful as an adjunctive therapy in controlling nausea and vomiting in some patients with gastroparesis.

ANTIEMETICS

The use of antiemetic medications is very common in clinical practice. Antiemetics are effective therapies for acute nausea and vomiting associated with chemotherapy, the postoperative period, and motion sickness. Antiemetics reduce vomiting by acting on a diverse range of receptors in the peripheral nervous system and CNS (**Table 2**). However, data supporting the efficacy of antiemetic agents in gastroparesis are very limited. There are no randomized controlled trials regarding the use of antiemetics in patients with gastroparesis, except for dopamine receptor antagonists, which also have prokinetic properties. Antiemetics should be used on an "as-needed basis" as an adjunctive therapy to prokinetics for the symptomatic control of nausea and vomiting. As with other pharmacologic treatment, the risk to pregnancies is also a factor in deciding on use (**Box 1**).

Phenothiazines

Phenothiazines are the most commonly prescribed antiemetics (see **Table 2**). They exert an antiemetic effect by blocking dopamine-2 and 5-HT receptors in the chemoreceptor trigger zone as well as having weak histamine-1 and muscarinic-1 receptor blocking activity. The most commonly used phenothiazines are promethazine (Phenergan) and prochlorperazine (Compazine). Promethazine is commonly dosed at 12.5 to 25 mg every 4 to 6 hours as needed. Promethazine is relatively inexpensive. Although it can be given orally, it can also be given as a suppository, intramuscular injection, and intravenous infusion. These alternatives to the oral preparation are useful in patients experiencing periods of severe emesis. Prochlorperazine is usually dosed at 5 to 10 mg every 6 to 8 hours as needed. Prochlorperazine can be given as oral tablets, intramuscular injection, and intravenous infusion (see **Table 2**). If prochlorperazine is administered via the intravenous route, it should be given as a short infusion (30 minutes) to avoid orthostatic hypotension.

Phenothiazines are effective therapies for acute nausea and vomiting associated with elective surgery, vertigo, motion sickness, and migraine, based on randomized controlled trials.[13–16] However, there are no data on the use of phenothiazines for chronic nausea and vomiting. Short-term, intermittent use of phenothiazines is a reasonable approach in patients with gastroparesis, but frequent use or high doses of phenothiazines should be avoided. Phenothiazines penetrate the CNS and frequently cause drowsiness, sedation, and confusion. Patients should be warned against driving, operating machinery, and strenuous activity. Concurrent intake of alcohol and other sedatives should be avoided. Lower doses of promethazine should be used whenever possible, especially in the elderly. Furthermore, both promethazine and prochlorperazine may cause extrapyramidal side effects, such as tardive dyskinesia and dystonia, due to their dopamine antagonism in the basal ganglia.[17]

Venous scarring with promethazine is a well-known adverse event. A Food and Drug Administration (FDA) patient safety bulletin has warned of the potential for tissue injury due to extravasation of intravenous promethazine.[18] Promethazine should be infused only through a large-bore vein, and the patency of the access site should be checked before administering. The patient should be instructed to report burning or pain during and after the injection. An intravenous port or peripherally inserted central catheter line should be considered if promethazine is ordered for home health use in patients with recurring nausea and vomiting.

5-Hydroxytryptamine 3 Antagonists

In response to toxic substances and formation of free radicals, large amounts of 5-HT are released from the enterochromaffin cells in the gastrointestinal mucosa. This circulating serotonin stimulates the 5-HT3 receptors in the chemoreceptor trigger zone within the CNS, resulting in emesis.[19] Pharmacologic use of 5-HT3 receptor antagonists exerts a diffuse blockade of the 5-HT3 receptors in the small intestine, chemoreceptor trigger zone, and nucleus tractus solitarius. The currently available 5-HT3 receptor antagonists in the United States are listed in **Table 2**. Genetic polymorphisms in the cytochrome P450 monooxygenase system, drug efflux transporter, and 5-HT3 receptor subunits may account for the variable interindividual response to the different 5-HT3 receptor antagonists.[20] Thus, it is reasonable to switch a patient from one 5-HT3 receptor antagonist to another, if the medication administered initially does not provide the desired symptom control.

The first drug of this class was ondansetron (Zofran), which is available in tablet, capsule, oral disintegrating tablet (ODT), and parenteral formulations. The 5-HT3 receptor antagonists are effective for acute vomiting associated with chemotherapy and vomiting after surgery based on randomized controlled trials.[21–25] However, this class of antiemetics is among the most expensive pharmacologic therapies for nausea and vomiting. There are no prospective data on 5-HT3 receptor antagonists for the treatment of nausea and vomiting associated with gastroparesis. Due to the lack of efficacy data in gastroparesis and their high cost, these medications should be used only in short courses and reserved for patients with refractory nausea and vomiting. The 5-HT3 receptor antagonists are generally well tolerated. Potential adverse side effects are headache, diarrhea, constipation, and dizziness. Although electrocardiogram changes have been attributed to 5-HT3 receptor antagonists as a class, serious cardiac events, such as torsades de pointes, have not been reported.[26]

Histamine and Cholinergic Antagonists

Antihistamines inhibit the action of histamine at the histamine-1 receptor, and anticholinergic agents inhibit acetylcholine at the muscarinic-1 receptor. These two classes of antiemetics block the stimulation of the emesis pathway that originates from the histamine- and acetylcholine-rich vestibular system. The currently available histamine and cholinergic receptor antagonists for nausea and vomiting are listed in **Table 2**. The advantages of these two classes of antiemetics include availability and formulation. Diphenhydramine (Benadryl), dimenhydrinate (Dramamine), and meclizine (Antivert) are available over the counter. Anticholinergic scopolamine is available as a transdermal patch by prescription.

Histamine and cholinergic antagonists have been shown to be efficacious in the treatment of acute nausea and vomiting associated with motion sickness and in the postoperative period.[27,28] As in other antiemetics, there are no randomized controlled trials of histamine and cholinergic antagonists in patients with gastroparesis. These agents are generally less helpful in gastroparesis, since the vestibular system does not play a prominent role in the pathophysiology of emesis associated with gastroparesis. However, the sedative and antiemetic properties of intravenous histamine antagonists may be helpful in hospitalized patients. The scopolamine transdermal patch may be useful in some patients with profuse vomiting who are unable to tolerate an oral antiemetic. Potential side effects of histamine antagonists are usually minor but include sedation, dizziness, fatigue, and tremor. The scopolamine transdermal patch

Table 2
Antiemetics Available in the United States

Antiemetic Class	Medications	Formations								Pregnancy Category[a]
		Tablet or Capsule	Suspension	ODT[b]	Trans-dermal	Suppository	Subcutaneous	Intra-muscular	Intra-venous	
Phenothiazines	Promethazine (Phenergan)	X	X	—	—	X	—	X	X	C
	Prochlorperazine (Compazine)	X	—	—	—	—	—	X	X	C
5-Hydroxytryptamine antagonist	Ondansetron (Zofran)[a]	X	X	X	—	—	—	X	X	B
	Dolasetron (Anzemet)	X	—	—	—	—	—	—	X	B
	Palonosetron (Aloxi)	—	—	—	—	—	—	—	X	B
	Granisetron (Kytril)	X	X	—	—	—	—	—	X	B
Histamine-1 antagonist	Diphenhydramine (Benadryl)[c]	X	X	X	—	—	—	X	X	B
	Dimenhydrinate (Dramamine)[c]	X	—	—	—	—	—	—	—	B
	Meclizine (Antivert)[c]	X	—	—	—	—	—	—	—	B
	Hydroxyzine (Atarax, Vistaril)	X	X	—	—	—	—	X	—	C
Cholinergic antagonist	Scopolamine	X	—	—	X	—	X	X	X	C
Dopamine antagonist	Metoclopramide (Reglan)	X	X	—	—	—	—	X	X	B
	Domperidone (Motilium)[d]	X	—	—	—	—	—	—	—	C

Butyrophenones	Haloperidol (Haldol)	X	X	—	—	—	X	X	C
	Droperidol (Inapsine)	—	—	—	—	—	X	X	C
Benzodiazepines	Midazolam (Versed)	—	X	—	—	—	X	X	D
	Lorazepam (Ativan)	X	X	—	—	—	X	X	D
Neurokinin-1 antagonist	Aprepitant (Emend)	X	—	—	—	—	—	X	B
Cannabinoids	Nabilone (Cesamet)	X	—	—	—	—	—	—	C
	Dronabinol (Marinol)	X	—	—	—	—	—	—	C
Others	Trimethobenzamide (Tigan)	X	—	—	—	—	X	—	C

a Pregnancy category descriptions provided in **Box 1**.
b Oral disintegrating tablet.
c Available over the counter.
d Available with an FDA Investigational New Drug Application.

Box 1
Food and Drug Administration Pregnancy Categories

Category A

Adequate and well-controlled studies have failed to demonstrate risk to the fetus in the first trimester of pregnancy, and there is no evidence of risk in later trimesters

Category B

Animal reproduction studies have failed to demonstrate a risk to the fetus, and there are no adequate and well-controlled studies in pregnant women

Category C

Animal reproduction studies have shown an adverse effect on the fetus, and there are no adequate and well-controlled studies in humans, but potential benefits may warrant use of the drug in pregnant women despite potential risks

Category D

There is positive evidence of human fetal risk based on adverse reaction data from investigational or marketing experience or studies in humans, but potential benefits may warrant use of the drug in pregnant women despite potential risks

Category X

Studies in animals or humans have demonstrated fetal abnormalities, and/or there is positive evidence of human fetal risk based on adverse reaction data from investigational or marketing experience, and the risks involved in use of the drug in pregnant women clearly outweigh potential benefits

---

can cause transient dry mouth and impairment of ocular accommodation due to its anticholinergic effects.[29] Drowsiness associated with the use of scopolamine is generally less prominent than that seen with the use of antihistamines.

Other Antiemetics

Several additional antiemetic agents warrant mention in the management of nausea and vomiting (see **Table 2**). Haloperidol (Haldol) and droperidol (Inapsine) are butyrophenones with dopamine-2 receptor antagonist activity. Haloperidol and droperidol are effective for preventing postoperative nausea and vomiting in randomized controlled trials.[30,31] The use of butyrophenones in the management of recurrent nausea and vomiting is limited due to potential side effects. Common side effects include anxiety, insomnia, and extrapyramidal symptoms. However, studies in patients with postoperative vomiting have shown that these adverse events can be minimized by using low doses, such as 1 mg of haloperidol intravenously.[32] Droperidol should be used with caution. The FDA has issued a "black box" warning on droperidol due to the potential of Q wave to T wave (QT) interval prolongation and torsades de pointes.[33] Cases of sudden death with high doses of intravenous droperidol have been reported; therefore, it is contraindicated in patients with a prolonged QT interval.

Midazolam (Versed) and lorazepam (Ativan) are benzodiazepines with some antiemetic and anxiolytic properties. They are useful in the treatment of acute and severe emesis associated with cyclic vomiting syndrome. Although data regarding the use of benzodiazepines in patients with gastroparesis are lacking, they may be considered in patients with gastroparesis who are hospitalized with nausea and vomiting.

Substance P is a neurotransmitter involved in many physiologic functions within the central and enteric nervous systems.[34] The Neurokinin-1 (NK-1) receptor, the receptor for substance P, is found within the vagal afferents peripherally and within the nucleus tractus solitarius and the chemoreceptor trigger zone centrally. Aprepitant (Emend) is a highly specific NK-1 receptor antagonist, which has been shown to be effective in preventing chemotherapy and postoperative emesis.[35,36] However, the high cost of both the oral and intravenous aprepitant limits its use, but it may be considered in refractory cases of nausea and vomiting.

Nabilone (Cesamet) and dronabinol (Marinol) are Drug Enforcement Administration–controlled scheduled class II and III medications, respectively. They are cannabinoids with antiemetic properties. In a meta-analysis of randomized controlled trials, cannabinoids were considered more effective than prochlorperazine, haloperidol, metoclopramide, and domperidone in the treatment of chemotherapy-induced nausea and vomiting.[37] However, dizziness, dysphoria, depression, hallucinations, paranoia, and hypotension are significantly more common in patients who received cannabinoids than the other antiemetics.[37] The use of cannabinoids should be avoided due to the chronic nature of nausea and vomiting associated with gastroparesis and the significant side effects associated with cannabinoids.

PROKINETICS

Medications with prokinetic properties have been used for decades. Prokinetics are the best studied pharmacologic intervention for gastroparesis, and they should be the mainstay of treatment in the majority of patients. The hypothesis of using prokinetics is that the symptoms of gastroparesis will improve by the acceleration of gastric emptying. However, gastroparesis is a very heterogeneous syndrome. The cause and effect relationship between emesis and delayed gastric emptying is difficult to prove. The number of currently approved prokinetics in the United States is limited, especially with the market withdrawal of cisapride and tegaserod.

Dopamine Receptor Antagonists

Dopamine receptor antagonists are the most commonly used prokinetics for gastroparesis and have been available since the early 1970s. The major advantage of dopamine receptor antagonists is that they have both prokinetic and antiemetic properties. Their mechanism of action is through the stimulation of gastric and upper small-bowel motility. Dopamine receptor antagonists also have an antiemetic effect in the chemoreceptor trigger zone, which is located on the blood side of the blood–brain barrier.

Metoclopramide (Reglan) is a central and peripherally acting dopamine receptor antagonist. It is available in tablet, suspension, intramuscular, and intravenous formulations. Intravenous metoclopramide in hospitalized patients with gastroparesis is an appropriate therapy. Subcutaneous injection of metoclopramide (10 mg/2 mL injection) has been described and can achieve serum concentration comparable to that of intravenous administration.[38] Metoclopramide at 10 mg orally before meals and at night is effective for the short-term treatment of diabetic gastroparesis in randomized controlled trials.[39–42] However, long-term maintenance therapy with metoclopramide has not been established by prospective clinical trials.[43]

The side effects of metoclopramide are common and numerous, including somnolence, reduction in mental acuity, fatigue, agitation, anxiety, and depression. These side effects are dose dependent, thus preventing the escalation of metoclopramide dosage beyond a total daily dose of 40 mg. Prolonged use of metoclopramide can cause Parkinson-like symptoms, which usually subside following discontinuation of the medication. However, tardive dyskinesia may occur with chronic use and may not reverse with discontinuation.[44] The patient should be informed of the potential side effects with metoclopramide, especially with chronic use.

Domperidone (Motilium) is a peripheral dopamine receptor antagonist with anti-emetic and prokinetic properties.[45] At high doses, domperidone is also a weak 5-HT3 antagonist, which may contribute to its antiemetic benefit. Unlike the multiple formulations of metoclopramide, domperidone is available only as a tablet. Domperidone is not available in the United States, but it can be obtained with an FDA Investigational New Drug (IND) application.[46] As a peripheral dopamine receptor antagonist, domperidone does not readily cross the blood–brain barrier, thus greatly decreasing the potential CNS side effects compared with metoclopramide. Domperidone is much better tolerated at higher doses than metoclopramide. Furthermore, domperidone can be used safely with minimal side effects in patients with Parkinson's disease.[47]

The efficacy of domperidone for diabetic gastroparesis has been demonstrated in multiple randomized controlled trials.[48–50] In a withdraw-design, multicenter, randomized controlled trial, 287 subjects with diabetic gastroparesis were treated with open-label domperidone 20 mg four times a day for 4 weeks.[49] A total of 208 subjects responded to this run-in period and were randomized to continue domperidone or matching placebo for 4 weeks. Upper gastrointestinal symptoms were significantly less in subjects who received domperidone. In a single-center experience with the FDA IND program, 192 patients were followed on open-label domperidone and were titrated up to a maximum of 120 mg/d based on symptom response.[51] Domperidone was effective in two-thirds of the patients, but only one-third were able to lower the dose or stop domperidone. The presentation and etiology of gastroparesis did not predict the efficacy of domperidone.

Similar to metoclopramide, domperidone increases prolactin hormone and can cause breast enlargement, breast tenderness, or galactorrhea in 3% to 11% of patients.[49–51] Patients with a history of a prolactin-releasing pituitary tumor should not receive domperidone. Cardiac electrophysiologic adverse events, such as a prolonged QT interval, have been described in animals treated with domperidone.[52] Cases of cardiac arrest have been reported in humans receiving high doses of intravenous domperidone,[53,54] leading to discontinuation of the intravenous formulation. Patients with ventricular tachycardia, ventricular fibrillation, and torsades de pointes should not receive domperidone. Male patients with a QT interval greater than 450 ms and females with a QT interval greater than 470 ms should be excluded from treatment with domperidone; therefore, an electrocardiogram should be obtained before initiation of therapy. The clinician should monitor for electrolyte disturbances, especially potassium, which may increase the likelihood of cardiac adverse events with the use of domperidone. With these precautions, the safety of oral domperidone tablets is supported by short- and long-term clinical trials.[49,51]

Motilin Agonist

Motilin is a gastrointestinal hormone secreted by the enterochromaffin cells in the mucosa of the stomach and duodenum. Serum concentrations of motilin consist of cyclical peaks corresponding to the initiation of phase III of the migratory motor complex (MMC), the "intestinal housekeeper" of the gut. This action propels undigested solids, such as raw vegetables and red meats, out of the stomach and into the duodenum. Motilin receptors are found directly on the gastrointestinal smooth muscles. Motilin's direct muscular contractile effect on the stomach is independent of cholinergic neural transmission.[55,56]

Erythromycin is a macrolide antibiotic with motilin properties at low doses. Although data are very limited, it has been suggested that other macrolides, azithromycin (Zithromax) and clarithromycin (Biaxin), may also have efficacy as prokinetic agents.[57,58] Erythromycin is available in tablet, suspension, and parenteral formulations. Erythromycin has a narrow therapeutic range as a prokinetic. The pattern and the extent of the erythromycin-induced phase III MMC contraction is dose dependent,[59] but not above 250 mg.[60] Erythromycin suspension is preferable in the outpatient setting, because it is more rapidly absorbed than the tablet formulation.[61] Erythromycin suspension can be administered at 100 mg to 200 mg three times daily 15 to 60 minutes before meals to obtain optimal postprandial prokinetic effects.[61] However, erythromycin suspension requires refrigeration and can be cumbersome for patients during the day.

Intravenous erythromycin is a potent gastric prokinetic in healthy volunteers and in patients with diabetic and postsurgical gastroparesis.[62–64] However, clinical efficacy data for oral erythromycin in gastroparesis are very limited.[55,65–67] Erythromycin is not an antiemetic, and its efficacy in reducing nausea and vomiting associated with gastroparesis is unclear. Long-term use of erythromycin is often limited by development of tachyphylaxis. If symptoms improve but relapse on erythromycin, it should be discontinued and can be reintroduced at a later date. Side effects of erythromycin may include nausea, vomiting, and abdominal pain, especially at doses above 250 mg. These symptoms often mimic the symptoms associated with gastroparesis.

Erythromycin is a macrolide antibiotic; therefore, it has the potential to prolong the QT interval. In a study of a state Medicaid database, the adjusted rate of sudden cardiac death was twice as high in patients who received erythromycin compared with that in patients who were not taking erythromycin.[68] This risk is further increased if the patient is taking medications that inhibit the CYP3A liver enzyme, such as ketoconazole, itraconazole, fluconazole, diltiazem, verapamil, cimetidine, clarithromycin, or troleandomycin. However, the doses of erythromycin in the affected subjects were not reported in this study.[68] Before prescribing erythromycin, it is essential to review each patient's current medication list. The cardiac risk is unclear for the smaller doses of erythromycin used for gastroparesis.

TRICYCLICS

Tricyclic antidepressants (TCAs) are used in the treatment of many functional gastrointestinal disorders, including non-cardiac chest pain, irritable bowel syndrome, and functional dyspepsia.[69] Stimulation of the stretch receptors by luminal distension is not affected by TCAs;[70] rather their efficacy is most likely a generalized dampening of symptom amplification in the CNS. Commonly used tricyclic agents for functional gastrointestinal disorders are amitriptyline (Elavil), imipramine (Tofranil), desipramine (Norpramin), and nortriptyline (Pamelor). It should be noted that the doses of TCAs used for this purpose are generally lower than the doses used for anxiety and depression.

The mechanism of action of TCAs in patients for nausea and vomiting is unknown. These medications have antihistamine and anticholinergic properties. The efficacy of TCAs has been shown in cyclic vomiting syndrome[71,72] and in functional unexplained nausea and vomiting.[73] In a retrospective review of 24 diabetic patients with nausea and vomiting unresponsive to prokinetic therapy, 88% reported at least moderate symptom improvement with open-label TCAs.[74] Of the patients, 68% reported that the TCA was the most effective therapy they had received. However, only half of these patients had delayed gastric emptying.

At this time, the benefit of TCAs for nausea- and vomiting-associated gastroparesis is unclear. The available studies of TCAs for other syndromes of nausea and vomiting consist of a small number of patients, and the studies are not randomized or controlled. TCAs should not be the first line of therapy in gastroparesis, but they can be considered in patients with significant dyspepsia. Common adverse effects of TCAs include sedation, agitation, and anticholinergic side effects. These potential side effects often lead to dose adjustments or discontinuation of the medication.

SUMMARY

Gastroparesis is a very heterogeneous syndrome. The cause and effect relationship between symptom generation and delayed gastric emptying is often difficult to prove. Multiple pharmacologic interventions are often needed in the treatment of nausea and vomiting associated with gastroparesis. Antiemetics reduce vomiting by acting on a diverse range of receptors in the peripheral nervous system and CNS. Antiemetics are effective for acute nausea and vomiting, but data are very limited regarding their efficacy in gastroparesis. They should be used on an "as-needed basis" as an adjunctive therapy to prokinetics. Prokinetics are the best-studied pharmacologic intervention for gastroparesis and are the mainstay of therapy. Domperidone is the most studied drug for the management of gastroparesis and has been shown to be efficacious in randomized, multicenter trials. Although not routinely available, domperidone is obtainable for clinical use. More research is needed to develop more effective pharmacologic and nonpharmacologic therapies in patients with gastroparesis.

REFERENCES

1. Parkman HP, Hasler WL, Fisher RS. American Gastroenterological Association technical review on the diagnosis and treatment of gastroparesis. Gastroenterologist 2004;127(5):1592–622.
2. Wo JM, Parkman HP. Diagnosis and management of functional dyspepsia and gastroparesis. Pract Gastroenterol 2006;30:3023–48.
3. De Block CE, De Leeuw IH, Pelckmans PA, et al. Delayed gastric emptying and gastric autoimmunity in type 1 diabetes. Diabetes Care 2002;25(5):912–7.
4. Jones KL, Russo A, Stevens JE, et al. Predictors of delayed gastric emptying in diabetes. Diabetes Care 2001;24(7):1264–9.
5. Maleki D, Locke GR III, Camilleri M, et al. Gastrointestinal tract symptoms among persons with diabetes mellitus in the community. Arch Intern Med 2000;160(18): 2808–16.
6. Ricci JA, Siddique R, Stewart WF, et al. Upper gastrointestinal symptoms in a U.S. national sample of adults with diabetes. Scand J Gastroenterol 2000;35(2):152–9.
7. Soykan I, Sivri B, Sarosiek I, et al. Demography, clinical characteristics, psychological and abuse profiles, treatment, and long-term follow-up of patients with gastroparesis. Dig Dis Sci 1998;43(11):2398–404.
8. Harrell SP, Studts JL, Dryden GW, et al. A novel classification scheme for gastroparesis based on predominant-symptom presentation. Gastroenterologist 2008; 42:455–9.
9. Wang YR, Fisher RS, Parkman HP. Gastroparesis-related hospitalizations in the United States: trends, characteristics, and outcomes, 1995–2004. Am J Gastroenterol 2008;103(2):313–22.
10. Quigley EM, Hasler WL, Parkman HP. AGA technical review on nausea and vomiting. Gastroenterologist 2001;120(1):263–86.

11. Del FA, Tonato M, Roila F. Issues in the measurement of nausea. Br J Cancer 1992;19(Suppl):S69–71.
12. Hornby PJ. Central neurocircuitry associated with emesis. Am J Med 2001; 111(Suppl 8A):106S–12S.
13. Sallan SE, Cronin C, Zelen M, et al. Antiemetics in patients receiving chemotherapy for cancer: a randomized comparison of delta-9-tetrahydrocannabinol and prochlorperazine. N Engl J Med 1980;302(3):135–8.
14. Baloh RW. Vertigo. Lancet 1998;352(9143):1841–6.
15. Wood CD, Stewart JJ, Wood MJ, et al. Effectiveness and duration of intramuscular antimotion sickness medications. J Clin Pharmacol 1992;32(11): 1008–12.
16. Pryse-Phillips WE, Dodick DW, Edmeads JG, et al. Guidelines for the diagnosis and management of migraine in clinical practice. Canadian Headache Society. CMAJ 1997;156(9):1273–87.
17. Skidmore F, Reich SG. Tardive dystonia. Curr Treat Options Neurol 2005;7(3): 231–6.
18. Severe tissue injury with IV promethazine. Available at: http://www.accessdata.fda.gov/psn/transcript.cfm?show=58#6. Accessed August 24, 2008.
19. Flake ZA, Scalley RD, Bailey AG. Practical selection of antiemetics. Am Fam Physician 2004;69(5):1169–74.
20. Ho KY, Gan TJ. Pharmacology, pharmacogenetics, and clinical efficacy of 5-hydroxytryptamine type 3 receptor antagonists for postoperative nausea and vomiting. Curr Opin Anaesthesiol 2006;19(6):606–11.
21. Crucitt MA, Hyman W, Grote T, et al. Efficacy and tolerability of oral ondansetron versus prochlorperazine in the prevention of emesis associated with cyclophosphamide-based chemotherapy and maintenance of health-related quality of life. Clin Ther 1996;18(4):778–88.
22. Hesketh PJ, Grunberg SM, Gralla RJ, et al. The oral neurokinin-1 antagonist aprepitant for the prevention of chemotherapy-induced nausea and vomiting: a multinational, randomized, double-blind, placebo-controlled trial in patients receiving high-dose cisplatin–the Aprepitant Protocol 052 Study Group. J Clin Oncol 2003; 21(22):4112–9.
23. Grimsehl K, Whiteside JB, Mackenzie N. Comparison of cyclizine and ondansetron for the prevention of postoperative nausea and vomiting in laparoscopic day-case gynaecological surgery. Anaesthesia 2002;57(1):61–5.
24. Johns RA, Hanousek J, Montgomery JE. A comparison of cyclizine and granisetron alone and in combination for the prevention of postoperative nausea and vomiting. Anaesthesia 2006;61(11):1053–7.
25. Watcha MF, Smith I. Cost-effectiveness analysis of antiemetic therapy for ambulatory surgery. J Clin Anesth 1994;6(5):370–7.
26. Navari RM, Koeller JM. Electrocardiographic and cardiovascular effects of the 5-hydroxytryptamine3 receptor antagonists. Ann Pharmacother 2003;37(9): 1276–86.
27. Wood CD, Manno JE, Wood MJ, et al. Comparison of efficacy of ginger with various antimotion sickness drugs. Clin Res Pr Drug Regul Aff 1988;6(2): 129–36.
28. Nachum Z, Shupak A, Gordon CR. Transdermal scopolamine for prevention of motion sickness: clinical pharmacokinetics and therapeutic applications. Clin Pharm 2006;45(6):543–66.
29. Schmid R, Schick T, Steffen R, et al. Comparison of seven commonly used agents for prophylaxis of seasickness. J Travel Med 1994;1(4):203–6.

30. McKeage K, Simpson D, Wagstaff AJ. Intravenous droperidol: a review of its use in the management of postoperative nausea and vomiting. Drugs 2006;66(16): 2123–47.
31. Tramer MR, Walder B. Efficacy and adverse effects of prophylactic antiemetics during patient-controlled analgesia therapy: a quantitative systematic review. Anesth Analg 1999;88(6):1354–61.
32. Wang TF, Liu YH, Chu CC, et al. Low-dose haloperidol prevents post-operative nausea and vomiting after ambulatory laparoscopic surgery. Acta Anaesthesiol Scand 2008;52(2):280–4.
33. FDA strengthens warnings for droperidol. Available at: http://www.fda.gov/bbs/topics/answers/2001/ans01123.html. Accessed August 24, 2008.
34. Otsuka M, Yoshioka K. Neurotransmitter functions of mammalian tachykinins. Physiol Rev 1993;73(2):229–308.
35. Navari RM. Aprepitant: a neurokinin-1 receptor antagonist for the treatment of chemotherapy-induced nausea and vomiting. Expert Rev Anticancer Ther 2004;4(5):715–24.
36. Gan TJ, Apfel CC, Kovac A, et al. A randomized, double-blind comparison of the NK1 antagonist, aprepitant, versus ondansetron for the prevention of post-operative nausea and vomiting. Anesth Analg 2007;104(5):1082–9 tables.
37. Tramer MR, Carroll D, Campbell FA, et al. Cannabinoids for control of chemotherapy induced nausea and vomiting: quantitative systematic review. BMJ 2001;323(7303):16–21.
38. McCallum RW, Valenzuela G, Polepalle S, et al. Subcutaneous metoclopramide in the treatment of symptomatic gastroparesis: clinical efficacy and pharmacokinetics. J Pharmacol Exp Ther 1991;258(1):136–42.
39. Perkel MS, Hersh T, Moore C, et al. Metoclopramide therapy in fifty-five patients with delayed gastric emptying. Am J Gastroenterol 1980;74(3):231–6.
40. Snape WJ Jr, Battle WM, Schwartz SS, et al. Metoclopramide to treat gastroparesis due to diabetes mellitus: a double-blind, controlled trial. Ann Intern Med 1982; 96(4):444–6.
41. McCallum RW, Ricci DA, Rakatansky H, et al. A multicenter placebo-controlled clinical trial of oral metoclopramide in diabetic gastroparesis. Diabetes Care 1983;6(5):463–7.
42. Ricci DA, Saltzman MB, Meyer C, et al. Effect of metoclopramide in diabetic gastroparesis. J Clin Gastroenterol 1985;7(1):25–32.
43. Lata PF, Pigarelli DL. Chronic metoclopramide therapy for diabetic gastroparesis. Ann Pharmacother 2003;37(1):122–6.
44. Ganzini L, Casey DE, Hoffman WF, et al. The prevalence of metoclopramide-induced tardive dyskinesia and acute extrapyramidal movement disorders. Arch Intern Med 1993;153(12):1469–75.
45. Reddymasu SC, Soykan I, McCallum RW. Domperidone: review of pharmacology and clinical applications in gastroenterology. Am J Gastroenterol 2007;102(9): 2036–45.
46. How to obtain domperidone?. Available at: http://www.fda.gov/cder/news/domperidone.htm. Accessed August 24, 2008.
47. Lertxundi U, Peral J, Mora O, et al. Antidopaminergic therapy for managing co-morbidities in patients with Parkinson's disease. Am J Health Syst Pharm 2008; 65(5):414–9.
48. Farup CE, Leidy NK, Murray M, et al. Effect of domperidone on the health-related quality of life of patients with symptoms of diabetic gastroparesis. Diabetes Care 1998;21(10):1699–706.

49. Silvers D, Kipnes M, Broadstone V, et al. Domperidone in the management of symptoms of diabetic gastroparesis: efficacy, tolerability, and quality-of-life outcomes in a multicenter controlled trial. DOM-USA-5 Study Group. Clin Ther 1998;20(3):438–53.

50. Patterson D, Abell T, Rothstein R, et al. A double-blind multicenter comparison of domperidone and metoclopramide in the treatment of diabetic patients with symptoms of gastroparesis. Am J Gastroenterol 1999;94(5):1230–4.

51. Wo JM, Woosley A, Eversmann J, et al. Open-label use of domperidone in patients with gastroparesis and small bowel dysfunction. [abstract]. Am J Gastroenterol 2008;103:546.

52. Drolet B, Rousseau G, Daleau P, et al. Domperidone should not be considered a no-risk alternative to cisapride in the treatment of gastrointestinal motility disorders. Circulation 2000;102(16):1883–5.

53. Roussak JB, Carey P, Parry H. Cardiac arrest after treatment with intravenous domperidone. Br Med J (Clin Res Ed) 1984;289(6458):1579.

54. Love EM, Yin JA, Delamore IW. Cardiotoxicity of intravenous domperidone. Lancet 1985;2(8456):676.

55. Bruley d V, Parys V, Ropert A, et al. Erythromycin enhances fasting and postprandial proximal gastric tone in humans. Gastroenterologist 1995;109(1):32–9.

56. Cuomo R, Vandaele P, Coulie B, et al. Influence of motilin on gastric fundus tone and on meal-induced satiety in man: role of cholinergic pathways. Am J Gastroenterol 2006;101(4):804–11.

57. Bortolotti M, Mari C, Brunelli F, et al. Effect of intravenous clarithromycin on interdigestive gastroduodenal motility of patients with functional dyspepsia and Helicobacter pylori gastritis. Dig Dis Sci 1999;44(12):2439–42.

58. Sutera L, Dominguez LJ, Belvedere M, et al. Azithromycin in an older woman with diabetic gastroparesis. Am J Ther 2008;15(1):85–8.

59. Tack J, Janssens J, Vantrappen G, et al. Effect of erythromycin on gastric motility in controls and in diabetic gastroparesis. Gastroenterologist 1992;103(1):72–9.

60. Desautels SG, Hutson WR, Christian PE, et al. Gastric emptying response to variable oral erythromycin dosing in diabetic gastroparesis. Dig Dis Sci 1995;40(1):141–6.

61. Ehrenpreis ED, Zaitman D, Nellans H. Which form of erythromycin should be used to treat gastroparesis? A pharmacokinetic analysis. Aliment Pharmacol Ther 1998;12(4):373–6.

62. Annese V, Janssens J, Vantrappen G, et al. Erythromycin accelerates gastric emptying by inducing antral contractions and improved gastroduodenal coordination. Gastroenterologist 1992;102(3):823–8.

63. Janssens J, Peeters TL, Vantrappen G, et al. Improvement of gastric emptying in diabetic gastroparesis by erythromycin. Preliminary studies. N Engl J Med 1990;322(15):1028–31.

64. Kendall BJ, Chakravarti A, Kendall E, et al. The effect of intravenous erythromycin on solid meal gastric emptying in patients with chronic symptomatic postvagotomy-antrectomy gastroparesis. Aliment Pharmacol Ther 1997;11(2):381–5.

65. Dhir R, Richter JE. Erythromycin in the short- and long-term control of dyspepsia symptoms in patients with gastroparesis. J Clin Gastroenterol 2004;38(3):237–42.

66. Richards RD, Davenport K, McCallum RW. The treatment of idiopathic and diabetic gastroparesis with acute intravenous and chronic oral erythromycin. Am J Gastroenterol 1993;88(2):203–7.

67. Samsom M, Jebbink RJ, Akkermans LM, et al. Effects of oral erythromycin on fasting and postprandial antroduodenal motility in patients with type I diabetes,

measured with an ambulatory manometric technique. Diabetes Care 1997;20(2): 129–34.

68. Ray WA, Murray KT, Meredith S, et al. Oral erythromycin and the risk of sudden death from cardiac causes. N Engl J Med 2004;351(11):1089–96.

69. Jackson JL, O'Malley PG, Tomkins G, et al. Treatment of functional gastrointestinal disorders with antidepressant medications: a meta-analysis. Am J Med 2000;108(1):65–72.

70. Gorelick AB, Koshy SS, Hooper FG, et al. Differential effects of amitriptyline on perception of somatic and visceral stimulation in healthy humans. Am J Phys 1998;275(3 Pt 1):G460–6.

71. Namin F, Patel J, Lin Z, et al. Clinical, psychiatric and manometric profile of cyclic vomiting syndrome in adults and response to tricyclic therapy. Neurogastroenterol Motil 2007;19(3):196–202.

72. Prakash C, Clouse RE. Cyclic vomiting syndrome in adults: clinical features and response to tricyclic antidepressants. Am J Gastroenterol 1999;94(10):2855–60.

73. Prakash C, Lustman PJ, Freedland KE, et al. Tricyclic antidepressants for functional nausea and vomiting: clinical outcome in 37 patients. Dig Dis Sci 1998; 43(9):1951–6.

74. Sawhney MS, Prakash C, Lustman PJ, et al. Tricyclic antidepressants for chronic vomiting in diabetic patients. Dig Dis Sci 2007;52(2):418–24.

Treatment of Refractory Gastroparesis: Gastric and Jejunal Tubes, Botox, Gastric Electrical Stimulation, and Surgery

Reza A. Hejazi, MD, Richard W. McCallum, MD, FACP, FACG*

KEYWORDS

- Refractory gastroparesis • Treatment • Prokinetics
- Enteral nutrition • Gastric neurostimulation
- Gastrectomy

Gastroparesis is a disorder characterized by a spectrum of recognized symptoms with evidence for gastric retention in the absence of mechanical obstruction. The range of symptoms includes nausea, vomiting, early satiety, and postprandial fullness. Abdominal discomfort and pain are also noted by some patients. It can be complicated by weight loss, malnutrition, dehydration, and electrolyte abnormalities in moderate to severe cases.

Published data have not identified the true prevalence of gastroparesis, but up to 7% of the United States population has been suggested to have some symptoms of gastroparesis. It affects women more than men with a female-to-male ratio of 4:1, and the mean age of onset is 34 years. The most common systemic disease associated with gastroparesis is diabetes mellitus. It is estimated that up to 5 million diabetic patients (combining type 1 and type 2) have gastroparesis in the United States alone based on a population estimate of 23 million diabetics. Idiopathic gastroparesis has a similar population incidence. The subgroup of postsurgical patients undergoing an abdominal or thoracic surgery (eg, Nissen fundoplication) and accidental vagal nerve injury constitute the next common cause of gastroparesis with an estimated number of about 1 million patients affected.[1-4]

Department of Medicine, Center for GI Nerve & Muscle Function, Division of GI Motility, Kansas University Medical Center, 3901 Rainbow Boulevard, MS 1058, Kansas City, KS 66160, USA
* Corresponding author.
E-mail address: rmccallu@kumc.edu (R.W. McCallum).

Gastrointest Endoscopy Clin N Am 19 (2009) 73–82
doi:10.1016/j.giec.2008.12.010
1052-5157/08/$ – see front matter. Published by Elsevier Inc.

Treatment strategies are based on control of symptoms (particularly nausea and vomiting), improving delayed gastric emptying, and providing dietary and nutritional support to stabilize weight and correct nutritional needs. To control symptoms of nausea and vomiting and enhance delayed gastric emptying, prokinetics are regarded as first-line medication in gastroparesis. In this category, dopamine D2 receptor antagonists such as metoclopramide, domperidone (not available in the United States), and itopride (a dopamine D2 antagonist with antiacetylcholinesterase effects)[5,6] have been used with various degrees of success.[7]

Motilin receptor agonists act by accelerating antroduodenal contraction to improve delayed gastric emptying. Some macrolide antibiotics, such as erythromycin, clarithromycin, and azithromycin are potent motilin receptor agonists and accelerate gastrointestinal (GI) transit. Erythromycin in intravenous (IV) administration was the strongest stimulant of gastric emptying among prokinetics,[8] and up to half of the patients treated with the oral form also had symptom improvement.[9] Mitemcinal (GM-611), an orally active erythromycin-derived motilin receptor agonist, had promising results in diabetic gastroparesis in preliminary studies.[10,11] Recently, ghrelin, a neurohumoral transmitter secreted by the stomach and thought to play a physiologic role as a stimulant of food intake, has been successfully used parenterally in patients with diabetic and idiopathic gastroparesis.[12,13]

5-hydroxytryptamine 4 (5-HT4) receptor agonists are the other group of drugs with prokinetic properties in the GI tract. In this group, cisapride had promising results in controlling nausea and vomiting in gastroparesis but was withdrawn from the US market in 2000 due to its effects on prolongation of Q wave to T wave (QT) interval, resulting in cardiac dysrhythmias and sudden cardiac death.[14,15] Tegaserod, a partial 5-HT4 receptor agonist that had no effect on the QT interval,[16] did accelerate solid-phase gastric emptying[17] but was also withdrawn from use in 2007 because of unexplained cardiovascular ischemic events.

Antiemetics are effective in reducing nausea and vomiting related to gastroparesis and are most beneficial when used in combination with prokinetic drug therapy (**Table 1**).

Table 1
Classes of antiemetic drugs

Class of Agent	Examples
Dopamine D2 receptor antagonists	—
With prokinetic activity	Metoclopramide, domperidone
Without prokinetic activity	Prochlorperazine, trimethobenzamide, thiethylperazine
Serotonin 5-HT3 receptor antagonists	Ondansetron, granisetron, dolasetron, tropisetron
Tricyclic antidepressants	Desipramine, nortriptyline, amitriptyline
Muscarinic M1 receptor antagonists	Scopolamine patch or tablets (Scopace)
Histamine H1 receptor antagonists	Dimenhydrinate, meclizine, promethazine
Cannabinoids	Tetrahydrocannabinol
Benzodiazepines	Lorazepam
Neurokinin NK1 receptor antagonists	Aprepitant

MORBIDITY OF REFRACTORY GASTROPARESIS

Refractory gastroparesis is defined as gastric failure with refractory symptoms despite medical therapy, inability to maintain nutrition via oral route, and need for frequent emergency room visits or hospitalizations.[1]

In this setting, a variety of complications may occur, for example, dehydration and electrolyte disturbance, and a nutritional assessment to evaluate the need to initiate enteral or parenteral support may be necessary. A 10% loss of weight during 6 months is consistent with current definitions of significant malnutrition.[18] Specific deficiencies to consider are hypokalemia and hypomagnesemia, iron deficiency anemia, and iron storage depletion (particularly after partial gastrectomy); 25-OH vitamin D after long-standing gastroparesis or after partial gastrectomy; and B_{12} levels, particularly if small-bowel bacterial overgrowth is present.

MANAGEMENT OF REFRACTORY GASTROPARESIS

There is no consensus on management of refractory gastroparesis not responding to antiemetic or prokinetic therapy, and the latter is often limited by the development of intolerable side effects. In a previous study by our group of 146 patients with gastroparesis, 110 (75%) who initially failed oral metoclopramide or experienced side effects required discontinuation of the drug; 74% responded to use of another prokinetic agent (typically domperidone), whereas only 26% were refractory to all prokinetic agents. A good response to pharmacologic agents was observed in the viral and dyspeptic subgroups of idiopathic patients, those with Parkinson disease, and the majority of diabetic patients, whereas a poorer outcome after prokinetics was observed in partial postgastrectomy patients, those with connective tissue disease, a proportion of type 1 diabetic patients, and the subset of those with idiopathic gastroparesis dominated by abdominal pain and history of physical and sexual abuse.[3] Before moving to advanced therapy, it is crucial to ensure that gastroparesis is responsible for the symptoms as well as optimizing current therapy by combining prokinetic and antiemetic agents to maximal doses. After failure of all attempts at pharmacotherapy, placement of a feeding jejunostomy and/or venting gastrostomy can be considered. Newer therapies being evaluated are pyloric injection of botulinum toxin and gastric electrical stimulation (GES). Gastric resection remains as a last resort. All approaches are discussed in this review.

Nutritional Support

Initiating enteral nutrition or total parenteral nutrition (TPN) has to be considered if oral intake fails to provide caloric and fluid requirements in gastroparesis. TPN is not the preferred route when the small bowel is intact and often results in complications, such as infection, thrombosis and hepatobiliary complication, and steatosis. In situations of severe malnutrition when surgery is planned and there is generalized dysmotility including intestinal pseudo-obstruction, TPN can be indicated for a short-term use. Its cost and complications are unacceptable for long-term nutritional support.

Enteral nutrition is the preferred route to provide caloric and fluid needs in severe gastroparesis. **Box 1** summarizes our criteria for initiation of enteral nutrition supplementation.

A gastrostomy tube (G tube) may be used for venting of secretions to decrease vomiting and fullness. It can be placed endoscopically, surgically, or by fluoroscopy guide. Kim and Nelson[19] and Michaud and colleagues[20] in 2 nonrandomized, unblinded studies with a small number of patients (8 and 18 subjects, respectively) showed some gastric decompression and relief of nausea in their heterogeneous population with gastroparesis. Our experience is that G tube decompression is required only in

> **Box 1**
> **Criteria for initiation of enteral nutrition supplementation**
>
> 1. Severe weight loss, for example, unintentional weight loss >5% to 10% of usual bodyweight during 3 to 6 months
> 2. Repeated emergency department visits or hospitalizations for refractory gastroparesis requiring IV hydration and electrolyte replacement and/ or IV medication
> 3. Patient would benefit from a way to absorb medications
> 4. Overall poor quality of life due to gastroparesis symptoms

intestinal pseudo-obstruction patients but not in the usual gastroparesis setting. Infusion of liquid meals into the stomach via a gastrostomy is not safe because of the likelihood of exacerbating symptoms and risk of pulmonary aspiration in the setting of delayed gastric emptying.

Jejunostomy tube (J tube) placement is the most common route for enteral nutrition. It is usually placed by laparotomy or laparoscopy. Although there are limited reports of direct percutaneous endoscopic placement as well as expertise by interventional radiology, in our center, we change the tube to a button device (Mic-Key button, Kimberly-Clark Worldwide, www.mic-key.com) after 4 to 6 weeks because it is more convenient and cosmetically acceptable. Enteral feedings can be initiated 24 hours after J tube placement. Standard polymeric formulas with a caloric density of 1.0 to 1.5 cal/mL (eg, Jevity 1.5, Nutren 1.5 unflavored, Promote, or Isosource HN) are begun at low infusion rates of 25 to 30 mL/h and advanced by 10 to 25 mL/h every 4 to 12 hours until a high, but tolerable, caloric intake is achieved (usually around 100 mL/h). Liquid formulations of medications can be given through the jejunostomy followed by low-volume water flushes. When first administering enteral nutrition, jejunal feedings should be delivered continuously 24 hours a day for up to 2 to 3 days. Then it is converted to nocturnal infusions to free up the daytime hours for oral intake and to participate in normal daily activities. High-caloric formulas (1.5–2.0 cal/mL) can reduce volumes and nighttime infusions. Supplemental hydration with water may also be needed. It is important to remember the "rule of J tube feeding:" oral caloric intake should not occur when the J tube is running, because calories within the small bowel will inhibit gastric emptying and induce further nausea and/or vomiting.

If diarrhea occurs, slow the infusion rate and also consider small-bowel bacterial overgrowth. In patients with considerable weight loss, enteral feedings should be initiated more slowly to avoid refeeding problems such as respiratory failure and congestive heart failure.[1] The most common complications of J tubes are clogging and skin infection, which can be prevented by using a J tube of at least 14 F diameter and by regular flushing after administering medications and when not in use during the day. Routine skin care is recommended with hydrogen peroxide, cotton swabs, and/or bacitracin or other topical antibiotic ointments (eg, Neosporin).

Tube replacements are at approximately 6 to 12 months or when adverse issues arise. An extra Mic-Key button J tube should be kept at home, because if the J tube comes out, a new tube is needed within 2 to 6 hours to prevent the opening from closing. J tubes are effective in providing nutrition, fluids, and medications in the case of either normal or abnormal small intestinal motor function.[21,22]

Pyloric Botulinum Toxin Injection

Prolonged periods of increased phasic and tonic motor activity of the pylorus termed "pylorospasm" are postulated as one mechanism of delayed gastric emptying in gastroparesis.[23] Based on this, pyloric botulinum toxin (Botox) injection was considered to reduce pylorospasm. Botulinum toxin acts by binding to presynaptic acetylcholine terminals and produces blockade at the level of the neuromuscular junction, thereby preventing cholinergic transmission and promoting muscle relaxation. Its efficacy was studied in several small open-label trials (1–20 subjects) in diabetic and idiopathic gastroparesis.[24–30] The used dose was 80 to 200 units injected endoscopically in circumferential fashion at four to five sites into the pylorus (**Fig. 1**). Mean symptom improvement was 45% (range, 29%–58%), and gastric emptying improved an average of 42% (range, 33%–50%), lasting 1 to 3 months after injection. However, recent studies with more subjects (63 and 78 subjects) showed an overall response rate of 43% in one report,[31] and in another study response rates based on etiology were 55% for diabetic patients, 51% for idiopathic patients, and 44% for those with postsurgical gastroparesis.[32] The latter study showed more favorable response rates in higher doses (150–200 units). In two placebo-controlled randomized trials from the same institution, improvement in gastric emptying, but not in symptoms, compared with placebo was shown in one study (n = 12)[33] after botulinum injection, whereas no improvement was observed either in symptoms or in emptying rates over placebo in the latter (n = 23).[34] In a recent double-blind, placebo-controlled trial, 32 patients were randomized to receive botulinum toxin A or placebo. After a 1-month follow-up, symptom improvement was achieved in 37.5% and 56.3% of botulinum and control groups, respectively. Although improvement in gastric emptying was observed in the botulinum group, it was not superior to that in placebo.[35]

Also, its short duration of action and need for repeated injection are other limitations of this approach. Based on this literature, we cannot recommended Botox in diabetic and idiopathic patients.

Gastric Electrical Stimulation

GES is an approach for refractory gastroparesis that has been approved and initiated for the past 10 years. The US Food and Drug Administration approved a high-frequency, low-energy GES (Enterra Therapy System, Medtronic, Minneapolis, Minnesota) in

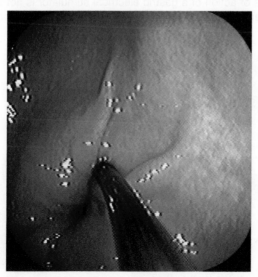

Fig. 1. Endoscopically guided botulinum toxin (Botox) injection into pylorus for gastroparesis.

March 2000 under a Humanitarian Device Exemption for symptomatic relief in patients with diabetic and idiopathic gastroparesis.[36] This system consists of a pair of electrodes sutured to the muscular layer of the greater curvature of the stomach 9 and 10 cm from the pylorus and is connected to a pulse generator implanted in a subcutaneous pocket in the abdominal wall. The pulse generator delivers low energy 0.1-second trains of pulses at a frequency of 12 cycles/min. Within each pulse train, individual pulses oscillate at a frequency of 14 cycles/s (**Fig. 2**).[1] Efficacy of GES has been evaluated in several studies, and for short-term follow up (1–12 months) the expected symptom improvement ranges from 15% to 93%.[36–43]

Our group investigated long-term results in 37 patients who had the device activated for a mean of 45 months. Total symptom scores, hospitalization days, and the use of medications were all significantly reduced at 1 year and were sustained beyond 3 years. At implantation, 15 of 37 patients required nutritional support and only five continued beyond 3 years. Mean HbA_{1c} level in diabetic patients was significantly reduced from 9.5% to 7.9% at 3 years.[44]

In May 2008 our center presented the results of up to 10 years Enterra therapy. In 46 of 93 (50%) of our patients who were available for a mean of 6.5 years (range, 5–9.5 years) of follow-up, the mean severity of GI symptoms decreased from 20 to 7 points (P<.001), and their mean frequency also decreased from 21 to 8 points (P<.001). Weight remained stable at 62 versus 71 kg. Mean HbA_{1c} level in diabetic patients was reduced from 8.9 to 7.9. A 40% reduction in gastroparesis-specific medication use was documented. Hospitalized days significantly decreased from 43 to 2.3 (P<.001). 70% reported near-complete relief of gastroparesis symptoms (>70% improvement). Complications were also identified: 27 (13%) patients underwent removal of device, 13 showed no improvement, two decided on removal as their symptoms completely resolved, seven had infection at the pulse generator site, two had small-bowel obstruction, two had protrusion of device through the skin, and one had electrode perforated to the lumen of the stomach. Nine patients required revision of systems due to electrode dislodgement related to trauma and/or twisting of connecting leads.[45,46]

The entire mode of action of a gastric electrical stimulator is not fully understood. Most studies observed a minimal or no acceleration in gastric emptying.[38,42,43,47–49]

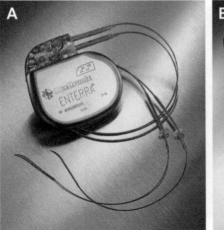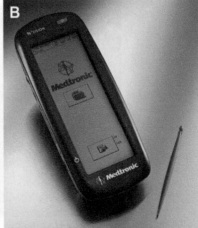

Fig. 2. Enterra system components. (*A*) Pulse generator. (*B*) Programmer.

Other possible mechanisms of actions are modulation of gastric biomechanical properties that enhance postprandial proximal gastric accommodation and reduce sensitivity to gastric distension;[50,51] inhibitory action of GES on afferent pathways projecting to different regions in the brain based on positron emission tomography;[52] and increase in vagal or cholinergic function as postulated in some studies.[53,54] However, understanding the exact mode of action of GES will require more investigations.

Surgery

Surgery is the last therapeutic option to be considered, and then only in a carefully selected subset of gastroparesis patients. The most common approaches include drainage procedures, such as pyloromyotomy or pyloroplasty, and bypassing a severely delayed stomach, such as partial or total gastric resections. Very limited data from uncontrolled reports show a small improvement in symptoms in pyloromyotomy or pyloroplasty.[55–57] Total and subtotal gastrectomy have been more effective, especially in post-antrectomy gastroparesis, in reducing symptoms and enhancing delayed gastric emptying.[58–60] We studied a series of nine gastroparetic patients (six diabetic patients with a fully intact stomach and three post-anterectomy) who underwent total gastrectomy with an average follow-up of 3.5 years (range, 1–5 years). Of the nine patients, six were available for follow-up (two died from renal complications of diabetes, and one was unavailable for follow-up). Hospitalization or emergency department visits were significantly reduced. In all patients, nausea and vomiting improved on average 55% (range, 40%–80%), and all were nutritionally stable with an accompanying J tube. Quality of life by their estimation had improved by 45% to 50% after total gastrectomy.[61] The main incentive to consider a total gastrectomy and esophagojejunostomy is to allow patients to stop vomiting and, hence, stay out of hospital and enhance their quality of life. Abdominal pain and the need for narcotics and other medications will still continue if they were present before the gastrectomy.

SUMMARY

GES is the major advance in this field in the past 10 years, offering new hope to this patient population. Radical surgery with subtotal- and total gastrectomy and feeding jejunostomy for backup nutrition and medications is reserved for patients not responding to the gastric stimulation therapy.

REFERENCES

1. Abell TL, Bernstein RK, Cutts T, et al. Treatment of gastroparesis: a multidisciplinary clinical review. Neurogastroenterol Motil 2006;18:263–83, 2.
2. Parkman HP, Hasler WL, Fisher RS. American Gastroenterological Association technical review on the diagnosis and treatment of gastroparesis. Gastroenterology 2004;127:1592–622.
3. Soykan I, Sivri B, Sarosiek I, et al. Demography, clinical characteristics, psychological and abuse profiles, treatment, and long-term follow up of patients with gastroparesis. Dig Dis Sci 1998;43:2398–404.
4. Patrick A, Epstein O. Review article: gastroparesis. Aliment Pharmacol Ther 2008; 27:724–40.
5. Holtmann G, Talley NJ, Liebregts T, et al. A placebo-controlled trial of itopride in functional dyspepsia. N Engl J Med 2006;354(8):832–40.

6. Stevens JE, Russo A, Maddox AF, et al. Effect of itopride on gastric emptying in longstanding diabetes mellitus. Neurogastroenterol Motil 2008;20(5): 456–63.
7. Sturm A, Holtmann G, Goebell H, et al. Prokinetics in patients with gastroparesis: a systematic analysis. Digestion 1999;60:422–7.
8. Kendall BJ, Chakravarti A, Kendall, et al. The effect of intravenous erythromycin on solid meal gastric emptying in patients with chronic symptomatic postvagotomy antrectomy gastroparesis. Aliment Pharmacol Ther 1997;11:381–5.
9. Richards RD, Davenport K, McCallum RW. The treatment of idiopathic and diabetic gastroparesis with acute intravenous and chronic oral erythromycin. Am J Gastroenterol 1993;88:203–7.
10. Ozaki K, Monnai M, Onoma M, et al. Effects of mitemcinal (GM-611), an orally active erythromycin-derived prokinetic agent, on delayed gastric emptying and postprandial glucose in a new minipig model of diabetes. J Diabet Complications 2008;22:339–47.
11. McCallum RW, Rogel R, Fang JC, et al. Mitemacil fumarate (GM-611) provided symptomatic relief of diabetic gastroparesis, especially in type 1 diabetics: results of a 12-week, multi-center, double- blind, placebo-controlled, randomized phase 2b study. Gastroenterology 2005;128:A467 [abstract].
12. Murray CD, Martin NM, Patterson M, et al. Ghrelin enhances gastric emptying in diabetic gastroparesis: a double-blind, placebo-controlled, cross-over study. Gut 2005;54:1693–8.
13. Tack J, Depoortere I, Bisschops R, et al. Influence of ghrelin on gastric emptying and meal-related symptoms in idiopathic gastroparesis. Aliment Pharmacol Ther 2005;22:847–53.
14. Abell TL, Camilleri M, DiMagno EP, et al. Long-term efficacy of oral cisapride in symptomatic upper gut dysmotility. Dig Dis Sci 1991;36:616–20.
15. Jones MP. Access options for withdrawn motility-modifying agents. Am J Gastroenterol 2002;97:2184–8.
16. Morganroth J, Ruegg PC, Dunger-Baldauf C, et al. Tegaserod, a 5-hydroxytryptamine type 4 receptor partial agonist, is devoid of electrocardiographic effects. Am J Gastroenterol 2002;97:2321–7.
17. Tougas G, Chen Y, Luo D, et al. Tegaserod improves gastric emptying in patients with gastroparesis and dyspeptic symptoms. Gastroenterology 2003;124:A54 [abstract].
18. Shopbell JM, Hopkins B, Shronts EP. Nutrition screening and assessment. In: Gottschlich M, editor. The science and practice of nutrition support: a case-based core curriculum. Dubuque (IA): Kendall/Hunt; 2001; p. 119–30.
19. Kim CH, Nelson DK. Venting percutaneous gastrostomy in the treatment of refractory idiopathic gastroparesis. Gastrointest Endosc 1998;47:67–70.
20. Michaud L, Guimber D, Carpentier B, et al. Gastrostomy as a decompression technique in children with chronic gastrointestinal obstruction. J Pediatr Gastroenterol Nutr 2001;32:82–5.
21. Fontana RJ, Barnett JL. Jejunostomy tube placement in refractory diabetic gastroparesis: a retrospective review. Am J Gastroenterol 1996;91:2174–8.
22. Jacober SJ, Narayan A, Stroedel WE, et al. Jejunostomy feeding in the management of gastroparesis diabeticorum. Diabetes Care 1986;9:217–9.
23. Mearin F, Camilleri M, Malagelada JR. Pyloric dysfunction in diabetics with recurrent nausea and vomiting. Gastroenterology 1986;90:1919–25.

24. Sharma VK, Glassman SB, Howden CW, et al. Pyloric intrasphincteric botulinum toxin (Botox) improved symptoms and gastric emptying in a patient with diabetic gastroparesis [abstract]. Am J Gastroenterol 1998;93:456.

25. Lacy BE, Schettler-Duncan VA, Crowell MD. The treatment of diabetic gastroparesis with botulinum toxin [abstract]. Am J Gastroenterol 2000;95:2455–6.

26. Muddasani P, Ismail-Beigi F. Diabetic gastroparesis a possible new indication for botulinum toxin injection [abstract]. Am J Gastroenterol 2001;97:S255.

27. Ezzeddine D, Jit R, Katz N, et al. Pyloric injection of botulinum toxin for treatment of diabetic gastroparesis. Gastrointest Endosc 2002;55:920–3.

28. Lacy BE, Zayat EN, Crowell MD, et al. Botulinum toxin for the treatment of gastroparesis: a preliminary report. Am J Gastroenterol 2002;97:1548–52.

29. Miller LS, Szych GA, Kantor SB, et al. Treatment of idiopathic gastroparesis with injection of botulinum toxin into the pyloric sphincter muscle. Am J Gastroenterol 2002;97:1653–60.

30. Arts J, Van Gool S, Caenepeel P, et al. Effect of intrapyloric injection of Botulinum toxin on gastric emptying and meal-related symptoms in gastroparesis. Gastroenterology 2003;124:A53.

31. Bromer MQ, Friedenberg F, Miller LS, et al. Endoscopic pyloric injection of botulinum toxin A for treatment of refractory gastroparesis. Gastrointest Endosc 2005;61:833–9.

32. Coleski R, Hasler W. Clinical and gastric functional predictors of symptom response to pyloric injection of botulinum toxin in patients with gastroparesis. Neurogastroenterol Motil 2005;17:628 [abstract].

33. Arts J, Caenepeel P, Degreef T, et al. Randomised double-blind cross-over study evaluating the effect of intrapyloric injection of botulinum toxin on gastric emptying and symptoms in patients with gastroparesis. Gastroenterology 2005;128:A544.

34. Arts J, Holvoet L, Caenepeel P, et al. Clinical trial: a randomized-controlled cross-over study of intrapyloric injection of botulinum toxin in gastroparesis. Aliment Pharmacol Ther 2007;26(9):1251–8.

35. Friedenberg FK, Palit A, Parkman HP, et al. Botulinum toxin A for the treatment of delayed gastric emptying. Am J Gastroenterol 2008;103:416–23.

36. US Food and Drug Administration. H990014—EnterraTM therapy system (formerly named gastric electrical stimulation (GES) system). March 31, 2000. Available at: http://www.fda.gov/cdrh/ode/H990014sum.html. Accessed March 31, 2000.

37. Familoni BO, Abell TL, Voeller G, et al. Electrical stimulation at a frequency higher than basal rate in human stomach. Dig Dis Sci 1997;42:885–91.

38. McCallum RW, Chen JDZ, Lin Z, et al. Gastric pacing improves emptying and symptoms in patients with gastroparesis. Gastroenterology 1998;114:456–61.

39. Forster J, Sarosiek I, Delcore R, et al. Gastric pacing is a new surgical treatment for gastroparesis. Am J Surg 2001;182:676–81.

40. Sobrino MA, Patterson DJ, Thirlby RC. Health-related quality of life with gastric electrical stimulation for gastroparesis [abstract]. Am J Gastroenterol 2002;97:S57.

41. Skole KS, Panganamamula KV, Bromer MQ, et al. Efficacy of gastric electrical stimulation for gastroparesis refractory to medical therapy: a single center experience [abstract]. Am J Gastroenterol 2002;97:S48.

42. Abell TL, Van Cutsem E, Abrahamsson H, et al. Gastric electrical stimulation in intractable symptomatic gastroparesis. Digestion 2002;66:204–12.

43. Abell T, McCallum R, Hocking M, et al. Gastric electrical stimulation for medically refractory gastroparesis. Gastroenterology 2003;125:421–8.

44. Lin Z, Sarosiek I, Forster J, et al. Symptom responses, long-term outcomes and adverse events beyond 3 years of high-frequency gastric electrical stimulation for gastroparesis. Neurogastroenterol Motil 2006;18(1):18–27.
45. Sarosiek I, Roeser K, Forster J, et al. A clinical outcome analysis of gastric electrical stimulation therapy (Enterra) beyond 5 years for severe gastroparesis, a single center experience. Gastroenterology 2008;134(4):A-535.
46. Sarosiek I, Forster J, Roeser K, et al. The incidence, spectrum and management of complications encountered during 10 years experience with Enterra therapy for the treatment of severe gastroparesis. Gastroenterology 2008;134(4):A468.
47. Lin Z, Hou Q, Sarosiek I, et al. Association between changes in symptoms and gastric emptying in gastroparetic patients treated with gastric electrical stimulation. Neurogastroenterol Motil 2008;20(5):464–70.
48. Lin Z, Forster J, Sarosiek I, et al. Treatment of gastroparesis by high-frequency gastric electrical stimulation. Diabetes Care 2004;27:1071–6.
49. Lin Z, McElhinney C, Sarosiek I, et al. Chronic gastric electrical stimulation for gastroparesis reduces the use of prokinetic and/or antiemetic medications and the need for hospitalizations. Dig Dis Sci 2005;50:1328–34.
50. Tack J, Coulie B, Van Custem E, et al. The influence of gastric electrical stimulation on proximal gastric motor and sensory function in severe idiopathic gastroparesis. Gastroenterology 1999;116:G4733 [abstract].
51. Cocjin J, Lin Z, Scoggan R, et al. Effects of high-frequency low-energy gastric electrical stimulation (Enterra device) on gastric distention and tone in gastroparetic patients. Gastroenterology 2005;128:A136 [abstract].
52. McCallum RW, Dusing R, McMillin C, et al. Fluoro-deoxyglucose (FDG) positron emission tomography (PET) in gastroparetic patients before and during gastric electrical stimulation (GES). Gastroenterol 2005;128:A622 [abstract].
53. Abell T, Lou J, Tabaa M, et al. Gastric electrical stimulation for gastroparesis improves nutritional parameters at short, intermediate, and long-term follow up. J Parenter Enteral Nutr 2003;98:277–81.
54. Lin Z, Cocjin J, Sarosiek I, et al. Influence of high-frequency electrical stimulation on gastric electrical activity, autonomic function and symptoms in gastroparetic patients. Neurogastroenterol Motil 2005;17:480–1.
55. Wooten RL, Meriweather TW. Diabetic gastric atony: a clinical study. JAMA 1961;176:1082–7.
56. Roon AJ, Mason GR. Surgical management of gastroparesis diabeticorum. Calif Med 1972;116:58–61.
57. Sodhi SS, Guo JP, Maurer AH, et al. Gastroparesis after combined heart and lung transplantation. J Clin Gastroenterol 2002;34:34–9.
58. McCallum RW, Polepalle SC, Schirmer B. Completion gastrectomy for refractory gastroparesis following surgery for peptic ulcer disease. Long-term follow-up with subjective and objective parameters. Dig Dis Sci 1991;36:1556–61.
59. Eckhauser FE, Conrad M, Knol JA, et al. Safety and long-term durability of completion gastrectomy in 81 patients with postsurgical gastroparesis syndrome. Am Surg 1998;64:711–6 [discussion: 716–7].
60. Forstner-Barthell AW, Murr MM, Nitecki S, et al. Near-total completion gastrectomy for severe postvagotomy gastric stasis: analysis of early and long-term results in 62 patients. J Gastrointest Surg 1999;3:15–21 [discussion: 21–3].
61. Saridena PR, Saridena RA, Sarosiek I, et al. Is total gastrectomy a good option for refractory gastroparesis? One site experience. Am J Gastroenterol 2008;103:S58, A147.

Surgery and Sacral Nerve Stimulation for Constipation and Fecal Incontinence

Rodrigo A. Pinto, MD, Dana R. Sands, MD, FACS, FASCRS*

KEYWORDS
- Fecal incontinence • Constipation • Sphincterplasty
- Sacral nerve stimulation

Fecal incontinence and constipation are two colorectal diseases that have a high incidence requiring specialized treatment when medical options are exhausted.

This article briefly discusses the etiology, epidemiology, incidence, and pathology history of constipation and fecal incontinence, followed by a detailed review of the surgical options, including SNS.

FECAL INCONTINENCE

Fecal continence is a complex bodily function, which requires the interplay of sensation, rectal capacity, and neuromuscular function. Multiple factors, such as cognitive function, stool consistency and volume, rectal distensibility, colonic transit, anorectal sensation, anal sphincter function, and anorectal reflexes, can influence a patient's continence.[1]

Fecal incontinence affects approximately 2% of the population and has a prevalence of 15% in elderly patients.[2,3] This disorder is a debilitating condition that can be personally and socially incapacitating. Incontinence is considered complete when the patient loses control of solid feces and partial when the patient has inadvertent soiling or escape of liquid or flatus. Browning and Parks[4] proposed criteria to stage fecal incontinence as follows: A, normal continence; B, incontinence to flatus; C, no control to liquid or flatus; D, continued fecal leakage. Subsequently, many grading scales have been proposed, and most consider the frequency of incontinence episodes as the most important item. Some scales,[5,6] which included urgency, cleaning difficulty, use of pads, and impact on quality of life, are considered more complete. Many authors have proposed scales for fecal incontinence. The Cleveland Clinic

Department of Colorectal Surgery, Cleveland Clinic Florida, 2950 Cleveland Clinic Boulevard, Weston, FL 33331, USA
* Corresponding author.
E-mail address: sandsd@ccf.org (D.R. Sands).

Gastrointest Endoscopy Clin N Am 19 (2009) 83–116
doi:10.1016/j.giec.2008.12.011
1052-5157/08/$ – see front matter © 2009 Elsevier Inc. All rights reserved.

Florida (CCF) fecal incontinence scoring system, described in **Table 1**, is a validated tool that is commonly used.[5]

Fecal incontinence has multiple etiologic factors, such as previous operative procedures, childbirth, aging, presence of procidentia, trauma, irradiation, neurogenic causes, primary disease, congenital abnormalities, or idiopathic causes. Each of these causes requires specific management depending on the severity of symptoms, presence of sphincter injury, and improvement after medical therapy. The etiology of fecal incontinence can be stratified into two groups: patients with normal pelvic floor and those with abnormal pelvic floor.

Fecal Incontinence with Normal Pelvic Floor

Aging
Elderly patients with a long history of straining of defecation may have injury to the pudendal nerve, consequently neurogenic incontinence can occur.

Gastrointestinal pathologies
Diseases that cause chronic diarrhea, such as inflammatory bowel disease, amebic colitis, progressive systemic sclerosis, infections, lymphogranuloma venereum or laxative abuse, can cause local sensory disturbance, mucosal irritability, and/or interference in the sphincter mechanism, resulting in a loss of reservoir function of the rectum.

Irradiation
Extracavitary or intracavitary irradiation for the treatment of cervical, uterine, and prostate carcinomas results in various degrees of proctitis, which can lead to incontinence.

Neurogenic causes
Patients with myelomeningocele or any disease that affects the central nervous system (CNS) or spinal cord, such as trauma, neoplasm, vascular accident, infection, or demyelization disease can have incontinence resulting from disturbance of sensory and motor nerve supply.

Overflow incontinence and soiling
Usually associated with fecal impaction, which causes a sensation of fullness, liquid stools can pass around the impaction resulting in seepage of liquid stool.

Idiopathic incontinence
Patients with no sphincter defects or other anorectal abnormality suffer from idiopathic incontinence. Neuropathic changes in the internal sphincter and abnormal

Table 1
Jorge/Wexner (CCF) continence grading scale (0 = perfect and 20 = complete incontinence)

Type of Incontinence	Never	Rarely	Sometimes	Usually	Always
Solid	0	1	2	3	4
Liquid	0	1	2	3	4
Gas	0	1	2	3	4
Wears pad	0	1	2	3	4
Lifestyle modification	0	1	2	3	4

Never, 0; Rarely, <1/mo; Sometimes, <1/d, ≥1/mo; Usually, <1/d, ≥1/wk; Always, ≥1/d.

sensation in the anal canal and rectum have been proposed as potential mechanisms.[2,3] These findings suggest neurologic damage.

Fecal Incontinence with Abnormal Pelvic Floor

Anorectal surgery
Internal sphincterotomy,[7] fistula surgery, hemorroidectomy, manual anal dilatation, and sphincter saving procedures have been shown to affect the internal sphincter and the external sphincter with resultant fecal incontinence.

Childbirth
Female preponderance of fecal incontinence occurs at a ratio of 8:1 in relation to that in males. Childbirth, mainly vaginal delivery, is the most important factor associated with sphincter injury. The reported incidence of occult sphincter defects after vaginal deliveries varies between 7% and 41%.[8,9]

Trauma
Direct trauma or impalement can often disrupt sphincter mechanism. Surgical repair may need protective colostomy depending on the extent of the injury.

Congenital abnormalities
Imperforate anus and the subsequent repair can result in fecal incontinence.

Procidentia
Complete rectal prolapse or procidentia may chronically injure the internal and external sphincters.

SURGERY FOR FECAL INCONTINENCE
Selection of Patients

Before any invasive intervention for fecal incontinence, the surgeon should have a through understanding of the etiology of the condition. Appropriate medical management can improve symptoms in the majority of patients. If the symptoms persist despite aggressive efforts to improve stool frequency and consistency and strengthen the anorectal musculature, surgical intervention is warranted. Evaluation of the anal canal with ultrasound is imperative at this point. The presence or absence of an anal sphincter defect dictates the proposed course of surgical intervention and the available treatment options.

Overlapping Sphincteroplasty

Disruption of the external anal sphincter, most commonly from childbirth or other forms of anorectal trauma, is repaired with the technique of sphincteroplasty.

The most common technique is the overlapping repair, first applied by Fang and colleagues,[10] Parks and McPartlin.[11] A transverse incision is made in the perineum, anterior to the anal canal. Lateral dissection allows for identification of the external anal sphincter muscle. Medial dissection is then performed to identify and preserve the existing scar tissue. An anterior levatorplasty followed by an overlap of the external anal sphincter muscle in the anterior midline is then accomplished. The scar is incorporated in the repair to strengthen the sphincteroplasty. **Figs. 1** and **2** show ultrasound images before and after the sphincter repair.

Early results were promising in 70%–80% of the patients.[12–16] Frequently, studies that reported better results were associated with a shorter follow-up, generally less than 3 years.[17–19] However, some others described poor results in a shorter follow-up

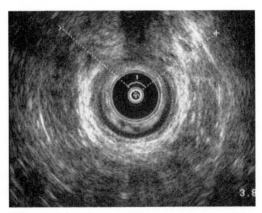

Fig. 1. Anal ultrasound showing anterior external anal sphincter defect.

period, ranging from 30% to 50%.[20–22] **Table 2** summarizes the success rates related to follow-up of the patients.

Tjandra and colleagues[32] conducted a randomized controlled trial comparing end-to-end and overlapping repair. Similar results were noted after follow-up of 18 months.

Use of fecal diversion to improve healing was reported by a recent prospective trial. Stoma-related complications occurred in seven of 13 patients.[33]

Recently published studies of the long-term follow-up after sphincteroplasty reported improvement of continence after more than 5 years.[26,30]

Repeated sphincteroplasty can be performed in patients who fail to improve in their continence and have a persistent sphincter defect. Success rates range from 50% to 65% in various studies.[34–36]

Postanal Repair

First described by Parks[37] in 1975, this procedure aims to reduce the obtuse anorectal angle and improve continence in patients with weak but intact sphincters.[38,39] Initially,

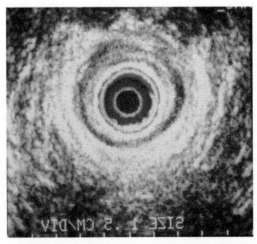

Fig. 2. Anal ultrasound after overlapping sphincteroplasty showing the external sphincter repaired.

Table 2
Short- and long-term results of sphincteroplasty

Author	Year	No of Patients	Follow-up (mo)	Results (Good or Excellent) (%)
FU < 3 years				
Osterberg et al[20]	2000	20	12	50
Malouf et al[23]	2000	55	12	76
Elton & Stoodley[17]	2002	55	13	80
Engel et al[18]	1994	55	15	79
Pinta et al[21]	2003	39	22	31
Norderval et al[22]	2005	71	27	41
Oliveira et al[19]	1996	55	29	71
FU >3 year				
Rothbarth et al[24]	2000	39	39	62
Morren et al[25]	2001	55	40	56
Grey et al[26]	2007	47	>60	60
Halverson & Hull[27]	2002	71	69	25
Zorcolo et al[28]	2005	93	70	55
Malouf et al[23]	2000	55	77	49
Barisic et al[29]	2006	65	80	48
Maslekar et al[30]	2006	72	84	95
Gutierrez et al[31]	2004	191	120	40

the dissection proceeds through the intersphincteric plane to the presacral space. Ileococcigeus, pubococcigeus, and puborectalis muscles are plicated followed by sphincteric plication.[38,39] The best results range from 76% to 81% success,[4,40] but most studies report more modest results with 31% to 68% success.[12] This modality of treatment is not commonly used.[41,42]

Injectables

Injectable bulking agents were initially used for urinary incontinence.[43] The first report on the management of fecal incontinence was described by Shafik[44] in 1993. The main advantage of its use is the ease of application, as it can be performed in the outpatient setting. Indications for injectables include passive incontinence, internal sphincter disfunction, and keyhole deformities. Several substances have been used for injection. Carbon beads (Durasphere), collagen, silicone, autologous fat, non-animal stabilized hyaluronic acid (NASHA-DX), and polytetrafluoroethylene, have all been described. None are currently Food and Drug Administration approved for clinical practice. Particles can be injected in the submucosal or intersphincteric plane, a place where less anal canal deformity is observed.

Collagen was injected into the submucosal plane under general anesthesia in 70 incontinent patients, showing a reduction of CCF incontinence score from 10 to 6 after 12 months of follow-up. The authors considered idiopathic incontinence and age above 60 years as predictors of success of the treatment.[45]

Tjandra and colleagues[46] injected silicon in the intersphincteric space in 82 patients. All retained the product after 1 month. After 6 months, all patients had significant improvement in symptoms and quality-of-life scale. While Maeda and colleagues[47] did not observe a significant improvement in incontinence score with long-term follow-up (61 months) of 6 patients, there was improvement in the quality of life of their social function scale. Silicone was also used for key hole deformities in 16 patients. Five patients had complete resolution of symptoms, and 11 had partial response after 1 year.[48]

Injectables appear to offer a safe, less invasive option for patients suffering from passive or mild fecal incontinence, which is persistent after conservative treatment.

Gracilis Muscle Transposition or Graciloplasty

Graciloplasty was described by Pickrell and colleagues.[49] The procedure uses the gracilis muscle to encircle the distal rectum and ultimately secure it to the opposite ischial tuberosity.

This is especially useful for patients with severe trauma or infection, which has resulted in significant tissue loss and destruction. The procedure is further modified by adding a nerve stimulator to improve the functional result.

Dynamic Graciloplasty

First reported by Beaten and colleagues,[50] the idea of stimulating the gracilis muscle with the implantation of a long-lasting pulse generator brought enthusiasm. The stimulation results in a change in types of muscle fibers from fatiguable to fatigue resistant, thereby allowing for sustained contraction.[51] A neurostimulator is implanted on the abdominal wall approximately 6 weeks after the gracilis transposition. The physician then adjusts the intensity of the stimulus. The patient turns the stimulator on and off to relax the muscles.

Dynamic graciloplasty improves the continence in 44%–79% of the patients. Twelve initial descriptions by Beaten and colleagues[52] showed good results, improving continence and quality of life of the patients.[53,54] **Table 3** demonstrates the results of dynamic graciloplasty for fecal incontinence.

Data from different authors suggest a high morbidity rate. Major related complications are infection (17%), stomal complication (25%), and evacuatory disfunction. Other less common complications, such as equipment dysfunction, perineal pain, and strictures occurred in less then 10% of the cases.[51] Matzel and colleagues[53] had a high incidence of complications in a prospective study with 121 patients, but all were treatable, and the overall recovery rate reached 87%.

Table 3
Results of dynamic graciloplasty

Author	Year	No of Patients	Continence Improvement (%)	Complication (%)	Follow-up (y)
Madoff et al[55]	1999	139	66	33	2
Baeten et al[56]	2000	123	74	74	1
Baeten et al[57]	2001	200	76	—	—
Wexner et al[58]	2002	115	60	—	2
Rongen et al[59]	2003	200	72	—	2
Koch et al[60]	2004	28	76	57 (32 expl.)	4
Thornton et al[61]	2004	33	60	—	5
Penninckx[62]	2004	60	78	73	4
Tillin et al[63]	2006	49	66	—	2

Expl., explantation.

Artificial Bowel Sphincter

First used to treat urinary incontinence, the artificial bowel sphincter (ABS)[64] was adapted for fecal incontinence by Christiansen and Lorentzen.[65] Patients eligible for the procedure usually have severe and intractable fecal incontinence resistant to other procedures or congenital anorectal malformations where their only option will be a permanent stoma.

Pelvic sepsis, Crohn's disease, scarred perineum, and perineal lesions induced by radiation are contraindications to ABS.[66,67] The procedure is performed under regional or general anesthesia with the patient in the lithotomy position. An anterior U-shaped perineal incision or two lateral incisions are made. A tunnel is created around the rectum for the placement of the cuff. After measuring the size of the ABS to be used, the sphincter is placed in position. The reservoir is placed in retropubic space through a suprapubic incision, and the pump is placed subcutaneously in the scrotum or the labia majoria. A radiopaque fluid is used to fill the three components of the ABS.[67] The cuff remains filled thereby closing the anus to achieve continence. The patient activates the pump to remove fluid from the cuff allowing evacuation. **Figs. 3** and **4** show the ABS before and after implantation. The success rates of ABS vary between 24% and 79%.[54]

Michot and colleagues[68] proposed the transvaginal approach for neosphincter implantation in women in 2007, showing 89% of success rate and only 11% of infection in 9 patients evaluated. Further studies are needed to prove the safety and efficacy of this approach.

The challenge of the ABS is infection. Placement of a foreign body in the anorectal region carries a significant risk of infection. The incidence varies, but the highest rates reach 40 to 60%.[12,54] Lower rates have been reported with a newer antibiotic regimen.[68] Erosion, ulceration, obstructed defecation, and chronic pain are other described complications. A multicenter cohort study investigated the safety and efficacy of ABS for fecal incontinence in 112 patients. Adverse events were reported by 99 patients, and there was a 25% incidence of infection. The explantation rate was 37%; however, 85% of patients with a functioning device had good outcomes.[69]

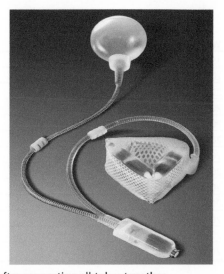

Fig. 3. System of ABS after connecting all tubes together.

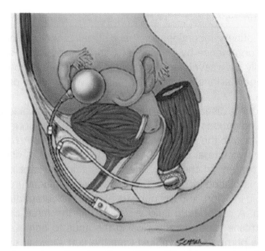

Fig. 4. ABS after implantation, showing the cuff involving the rectal wall, the balloon (reservoir) in the retropubic space, and the pump placed into the subcutaneous area of the greater lips.

Although it can be a challenge to avoid infection, if the surgery is successful, the ABS provides a viable alternative to stoma in carefully selected patients. This procedure should be reserved for patients with severe life altering incontinence and should be performed by experienced surgeons. **Table 4** contains the results of ABS.

SNS for Fecal Incontinence

SNS was first introduced in 1981 for urinary urge incontinence and obstructive urinary retention. Tanagho and Schmidt[82] noted that in some patients with dual incontinence, the bowel symptoms also improved. The first report of the use of SNS for three fecal

Table 4 Results of ABS						
Author	Year	No of Patients	Complication (%)	Explanted (%)	Success (%)	Follow-up (Months)
Cristiansenet et al[70]	1999	17	70	41	47	84
Lehur et al[71]	2000	24	17	29	75	20
Altomare et al[72]	2001	28	46	18	75	19
Wong et al[69]	2002	115	86	37	85	12
Ortiz et al[73]	2002	22	40	31	68	28
Devesa et al[74]	2002	53	57	19	65	26.5
Michot et al[75]	2003	37	—	24	78.9	>24
Parker et al[76]	2003	45	51	40	49	24
Da Silva et al[77]	2004	11	45	0	100	19
Casal et al[78]	2004	10	60	30 (20 rmpt.)	90	29
La Torre et al[79]	2004	8	25	25	75	3–40
O'Brien et al[80]	2004	7	42	14	86	6
Melenhorst et al[81]	2008	33	24	21	61	17.4

Rmpt., reimplanted.

incontinent patients was in 1995.[83] Since then, several studies have found this modality of treatment to be an interesting alternative to the treatment of fecal incontinence. The procedure is less invasive than the ABS, safe, and provides considerable functional improvement. **Fig. 5** shows the sacral nerve stimulator device in place.

There have been repots of SNS used in the treatment of fecal incontinence from a variety of causes, such as idiopathic sphincter degeneration,[84] iatrogenic internal sphincter damage,[85] scleroderma,[86] rectal prolapse,[85] partial spinal cord injury, and after low anterior resections.[87,88] Recently, it was proposed for treatment of fecal incontinence due to external sphincter defect less than or equal to 120°.[89,90] SNS has resulted in improvement in continence in 35%–100% of patients.[54]

SNS can be performed after failure of conservative management before other surgical procedures or even after unsuccessful surgical intervention. Another advantage is the test stimulation performed on an outpatient basis, which selects responders and nonresponders to the proposed treatment. Test stimulation consists of implantation of a tined electrode into the third sacral foramina. The electrode is attached to a percutaneous extension. A temporary generator is placed, and the response to a therapy is evaluated over a 2-week period. If a good response (>50% reduction in the number of incontinent episodes) is obtained, the percutaneous extension is removed, and a permanent stimulator is implanted. **Fig. 6** is a schematic view of the sacral nerve stimulator placed into the third sacral space and **Fig. 7** is a radiological picture.

The procedure has minimal morbidity, with complications ranging from 5% to 26%.[91] The most common complications reported are pain in the pulse generator site and superficial wound infection, ranging from 9% to 26% and 3% to 17%, respectively.[91,92]

The mechanism of SNS action on the pelvic floor muscles and colorectal transit is still unclear. Michelsen and colleagues[93] studied colon transit in 20 patients who underwent SNS and concluded that it reduces the antegrade transit through the ascending colon and increases the retrograde from the descending colon, which may prolong the colonic transit time and augment the storage capacity of the colon.

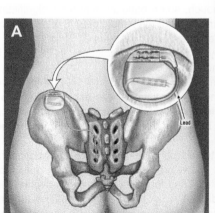
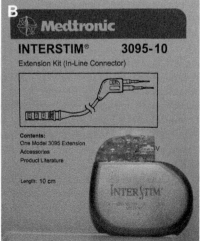

Fig. 5. (A) Sacral nerve stimulator (*Courtesy of* Dr. Badma Bashankaev). (B) System implanted in the patient.

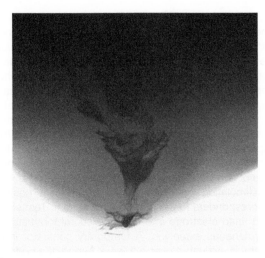

Fig. 6. Rectoanal intussusception.

Vaizey and colleagues[94] did a double-blinded crossover study with two women. The stimulator was on for 2 weeks and off for 2 weeks. When the stimulator was off, the patients' fecal incontinence worsened.

Chronic stimulation provides a good sensory effect, but the threshold is too low to induce motor effects. Some studies on fecal-incontinent and constipated patients demonstrated increased rectal sensation.[95,96] Holzer and colleagues[97] suggest that the stimulation of afferent nerve fibers of the rectal wall and pelvic floor have a positive impact on pelvic floor dysfunction.

Changes in cortical activity were noted in SNS patients in a study performed by Sheldon and colleagues[98] with 10 women. They concluded that SNS produces reversible reduction in corticoanal excitability leading to dynamic brain changes, which may influence anal continence.

The effects of SNS on rectal blood flow and autonomic nerve function was examined by Kenefick and colleagues[95] in 16 patients, finding a significant but reversible response, with a level of 1.0 V.

After low anterior resection or ileal J-pouch, some patients may have significant fecal incontinence. Some studies have demonstrated the benefit of SNS after anterior resection, but with a small number of patients and short follow-up.[97,99,100]

Permanent stimulation was achieved by 74.6%–100% of patients.[101–106] **Table 5** summarizes the results of SNS for fecal incontinence.

Symptomatic improvement greater than 50% was reported by 75%–100% of the patients who had permanent implant, and full continence was achieved in 40%–75%.[101,102,112–114] The majority of the studies used the CCF incontinence score, which showed significant improvement after 12 months. Quality of life was also improved after SNS.[85,102,104]

In 2008, Brouwer and colleagues[109] studied permanent SNS for 55 incontinent patients, comparing the efficacy of SNS in the presence of a sphincter defect or previous sphincter repair to intact sphincter. They found significant improvement in the median CCF score for all patients (median of 15 to 5) after 37 months. The authors also reported significant improvement in the four scales of quality-of-life score, with no significant difference between patients with sphincter defect or previous repair and those who have never had a sphincter defect. Altomare and colleagues[110] presented

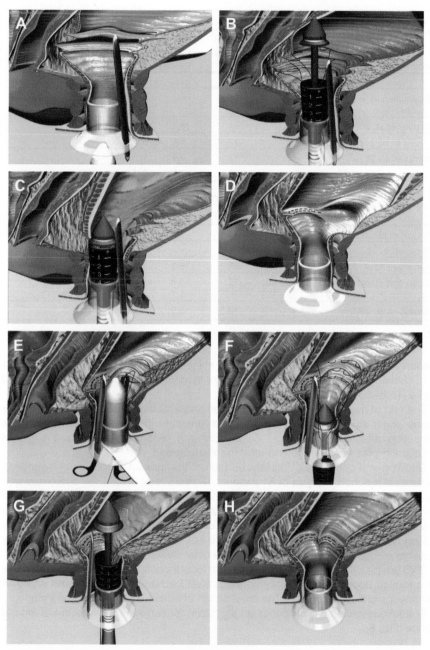

Fig. 7. STARR Procedure—insertion of the anal dilator to identify the rectoanal intussusception, followed by protection of the posterior rectal wall with a retractor. (*A*) Three sutures are placed in the anterior rectal wall 1–2 cm above the hemorrhoidal apex including the rectoanal intussusception; (*B*) The circular stapler is introduced, and its head placed above the 3 anterior sutures. Before firing the stapler, verify to ensure exclusion of the posterior vaginal wall; (*C*) Aspect of the staple line after withdrawing the circular stapler; (*D*) Repeat the same steps for the posterior resection, having at the end a full-thickness circumferential excision of the distal rectal wall (*E–H*).

Table 5
Results of SNS for fecal incontinence

Author/Yr	No of Patients	Follow-up (mo)	Incontinent Episodes/Week		CCF Incontinence Score	
			Baseline	Follow-up	Baseline	Follow-up
Rasmussen et al, 2004[107]	37	36	—	—	16	6
Matzel et al, 2004[105]	34	24	16.4	3.1	—	—
Uldag et al, 2004[108]	75	12	7.5	0.67	—	—
Jarret et al, 2005[100]	46	12	7.5	1	—	—
Hetzer et al, 2007[104]	37	13	7.5	2	16	5
Holzer et al, 2007[97]	36	35	7	2	—	—
Melenhorst et al, 2007[106]	100	25.5	31.3	4.8	—	—
Vitton et al, 2008[90]	5	14	7	2	15	6
Brouwer et al, 2008[109]	55	37	—	—	15	5
Altomare et al, 2008[110]	32	68	15.3	0.5	15.8	4.8
Chan and Tjandra 2008[111]	53 (21 SD, 32 NSD)	12	13.8 6.7	5 2	—	—
Jarrett et al, 2008[103]	8	26.5	5.5	1.5	—	—

Abbreviations: SD, Sphincter defect; NSD, Non-sphincter defect.

the long-term follow-up of 32 patients with at least 5 years after permanent implantation, showing a significant reduction in major incontinent episodes (15.–0.5) and CCF score (15.8–4.8).

The role of manometry in patient selection and evaluation treatment is still unclear. Some larger studies showed squeeze anal pressure increase and improved rectal sensation after SNS.[18,92,105,115] Others did not report any significant alteration comparing pressures before and after the stimulation.[91,108]

Dudding and colleagues,[116] analyzed factors that predict outcomes of incontinent patients in a cohort analysis of 81 patients 10 years after SNS. Their outcomes were not affected by patient age, gender, body mass index, and severity or length of symptoms. Repeated temporary procedure was associated with high incidence of failure in the screening. Better outcomes were observed when there was a lower threshold during temporary insertion. The authors did not find significant differences between patients with and without external anal sphincter defects.

SNS is a promising option for patients with fecal incontinence. It avoids implantation of a foreign body in a potentially contaminated field and affords patients improved continence and quality of life. The mechanism of action is still poorly understood.

The following diagram proposes an algorithm for surgical management of incontinence (**Fig. 8**).

CONSTIPATION

Constipation is one of the most common gastrointestinal disorders. In the United States, it is the cause of more than 2.5 million visits to physician offices, 3 million prescriptions of cathartics, and $800 millions spent on laxatives per year.[117]

The variety of symptoms and risk factors suggest a multifactorial origin. Connell and colleagues[118] in the 1960s evaluated the population of England and found 99% had

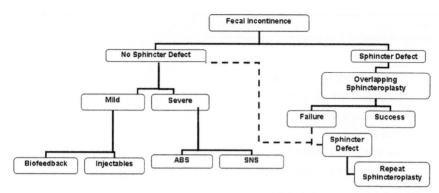

Fig. 8. Algorithm for surgical management of fecal incontinence.

bowel frequencies varying between three per day and three per week.[118] Since then, constipation is defined as having less than three bowel movements per week. Patients and physicians consider abdominal bloating and pain, straining to pass the stool, inability to defecate when desired, and hard stools symptoms of constipation.

In 2000, the Rome II criteria were proposed to define constipation. It consists of two or more of the subsequent abnormalities for the last 3 months: less than three bowel movements a week, sensation of incomplete evacuation, feeling of anorectal obstruction, hard or lumpy stool, straining, or need of manual maneuvers (digital disimpaction).[119]

Scales to measure constipation have been created. Wexner proposed a measure used to evaluate patients' improvement after clinical or surgical management (**Box 1**).[120]

Excluding the anatomic causes of constipation, such as neoplasms, strictures, adhesions, and extrinsic compression, all other causes are considered functional, as described in **Box 2**.

Lifestyle-Related Causes

Patients with low-fiber diet tend to be constipated. In addition, sedentary individuals and those who take medication that causes constipation, such as psychotropic drugs and opioids also tend to be affected. Laxative abuse can be another cause of constipation.

Metabolic

There are multiple endocrine states that lead to constipation, and they are listed in **Box 2**.

PELVIC OUTLET OBSTRUCTION
Rectocele

Herniation of the anterior wall of the rectum into the vaginal lumen (**Fig. 9**) is consequence of rectovaginal septum weakness. Multiple childbirths and advanced age are the main causes. Stools can be trapped in the herniation leading to incomplete evacuation. Physical examination reveals a rectocele in up to 81% of women, but only half of these patients have symptoms of constipation or difficulty of defecation.[121]

Box 1
Wexner constipation score (minimum, 0; maximum, 30)

Symptom (Score)

    Frequency of bowel movements

        1–2 times per 1–2 days (0)

        2 times per week (1)

        Once per week (2)

        Less than once a week (3)

        Less than once a month (4)

    Difficulty: pain evacuation effort

        Never (0)

        Rarely (1)

        Sometimes (2)

        Usually (3)

        Always (4)

    Completeness: feeling incomplete evacuation

        Never (0)

        Rarely (1)

        Sometimes (2)

        Usually (3)

        Always (4)

    Abdominal pain

        Never (0)

        Rarely (1)

        Sometimes (2)

        Usually (3)

        Always (4)

    Time: minutes in lavatory per attempt

        <5 (0)

        5–10 (1)

        10–20 (2)

        20–30 (3)

        >30 (4)

    Assistance: type of assistance

        Without assistance (0)

        Stimulant laxatives (1)

        Digital assistance or enemas (2)

Failure: unsuccessful attempts for evacuation in 24 hours

Never (0)

1–3 (1)

3–6 (2)

6–9 (3)

>9 (4)

History: duration of constipation (years)

0 (0)

1–5 (1)

5–10 (2)

10–20 (3)

>20 (4)

Agachan and colleagues (do constipation).

Descending Perineum Syndrome

Descending perineum syndrome is the result of the weakness of pelvic floor support, which is the consequence of sacral or pudendal nerve injuries or damage to the musculature itself during childbirth or chronic straining. Obstructed defecation occurs because of widening of the anorectal angle, weakening of the perineal body, and a vertical orientation of the rectum.[121]

Nonrelaxing Puborectalis Syndrome

Nonrelaxing puborectalis syndrome is also referred to as paradoxical puborectalis syndrome, spastic pelvic floor syndrome, anismus, levator spasm, and levator ani syndrome. Normally, with attempted defecation, the external sphincter and the puborectalis muscle relax, leading to strengthening of anorectal angle and facilitating evacuation. The failure of the puborectalis muscle to relax or paradoxical contraction causes continued maintenance of anorectal angle, effecting anal outlet obstruction. Puborectalis hypertrophy is the cause of anismus.[122]

Intussusception

Intussusception occurs when the proximal rectum is prolapsed into the ampulla but not through the anal canal (see **Fig. 6**). It is considered an early stage of rectal prolapse. Symptoms include difficult and incomplete sense of evacuation. Less commonly, pain, soiling, and incontinence are encountered.

STC or Colonic Inertia

STC or colonic inertia (CI) affects mostly women in the second or third decades. There is a strong association with gynecologic complaints, such as irregular menstrual cycles, ovarian cysts, and galactorrhea. Patients with slow transit constipation have a morphologically normal colon and rectum, but a reduced stool frequency.[123] Delayed gastric emptying, slow small-bowel transit, and biliary dyskinesia are commonly associated with STC, suggesting the presence of a pan-enteric motility disorder.[124–126] The evaluation of STC includes the assessment of colonic transit

Box 2
Etiology of functional constipation

Lifestyle-related causes

- Diet
- Pace of life
- Medications
- Weight loss/anorexia/laxative abuse

Infectious etiology

- Trypanosomiasis

Functional abnormalities with or without mechanical component

- Slow transit colonic constipation (STC)
- STC with megarectum/megacolon
- Obstructed defecation
  o Paradoxical puborectalis contraction
  o Intussusception
  o Descending perineum
  o Rectocele

Metabolic and other abnormalities

- Diabetes mellitus
- Hypotireoidism
- Hypopituitarism
- Porphyria
- CNS trauma
- Parkinson's disease
- Brain and CNS tumors

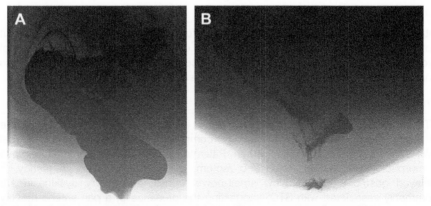

Fig. 9. (*A, B*) Anterior rectocele of 4 cm with significant retention of contrast.

with radiologic markers. Diffuse retention of the markers throughout the entire colon after the fifth day of evaluation constitutes slow transit constipation. Other systemic neuralgic processes, such as diabetes mellitus or multiple sclerosis, or a pelvic floor abnormality, should be excluded.

The initial management of constipation focuses on lifestyle and dietary manipulation. Increasing fiber and water intake as well as the addition of an aerobic exercise program will help the majority of patients with mild constipation symptoms. Exclusion of metabolic sources is an important step in the evaluation of this patient population. In patients who fail to resolve their symptoms with the above recommendations, an anorectal physiologic evaluation is appropriate. Defecography, surface electromyography, and transit studies are all used in the diagnostic armamentarium to determine the etiology of constipation.

SURGERY FOR CONSTIPATION
Selection of Patients

Before embracing any invasive treatment of constipation, it is necessary to determine the cause. It is the author's practice to address the lowest anatomic cause for constipation first. Pelvic outlet obstruction must be diagnosed and treated before any surgery for colonic transit alterations. The pelvic floor is investigated with defecography, magnetic resonance defecography, manometry, and electromyography. Patients with significantly decreased stool frequency warrant an evaluation of colonic transit as well. After completing the evaluation, the patient is categorized as follows:

1. Pelvic outlet obstruction
2. Slow-transit constipation
3. Combined STC and outlet obstruction

The goals of all surgical management of constipation are to increase the number of bowel movements and improve the quality of life of the patients.

Surgery for Pelvic Outlet Obstruction

Rectocele repair
Surgery for rectocele is indicated if the diameter is greater than 4 cm, there is evidence of nonemptying on defecography, and the patient has the appropriate symptoms. Co-existing conditions, such as rectoanal intussusception, sigmoidocele, and paradoxical puborectalis contraction can predict a worse outcome after surgical procedures, as the rectocele can be a secondary condition.[127]

Rosato[128] described criteria to select patients for surgery:

1. Rectocele >4 cm in diameter as measured by defecography
2. Non- or partial emptying of rectocele during push on defecography
3. Rectal or vaginal symptoms for longer than 12 months
4. Persistence of symptoms for at least 4 weeks despite increased fiber intake of up to 35 g/d
5. Need for vaginal or rectal digitations to facilitate evacuation

As least, three of these five criteria should be present. The approach for rectocele repair varies. Transvaginal, transanal, transperineal, or a combination of these have been described, with or without mesh.

Transvaginal repair
Transvaginal technique consists of opening the posterior vaginal wall, identifying the rectovaginal septum, and separating the anterior rectal wall to expose the levator

muscle. Sutures are placed in the levator muscle, plicating in the midline. Care has to be taken not to include the rectal wall or perforate while placing the sutures. The redundant vaginal wall is then excised and closed with absorbable running sutures.[129] An absorbable or nonabsorbable mesh can also be placed to reinforce the rectovaginal septum and avoid recurrence. The most common postoperative complications include pelvic pain and sexual dysfunction.[129–131] This is the technique most often used by gynecologists.

Transperineal repair
Transperineal approach is an option for repair of rectocele. The dissection is performed through the vaginal vault, and a band of the posterior vaginal wall is resected. The levator muscle is plicated in the same way as in transvaginal repair, and the vaginal wall is closed with absorbable running sutures. The mesh is also applicable.[132]

Transanal repair
Transanal procedures involve plication of the rectal muscular layer in a vertical or transverse fashion after resection of the redundant mucosa.[133,134,142] Different techniques have been proposed, such as simple obliterate suture[135] or stapling procedures, first described by Bresler and colleagues.[136] These vary from linear stapling to stapled transanal rectal resection (STARR) with a circular stapler.[137] Transanal approach is contraindicated in the presence of fecal incontinence because it is deleterious to the internal and external sphincter function.[138] Sullivan and colleagues[139] reported an early series of transanal rectocele repairs with 97.5% success in 150 patients. Their complication rate was low; however, there was one rectovaginal fistula.

A retrospective matched cohort study conducted by Thornton and colleagues[140] compared the transanal approach to laparoscopic repair, reporting better bowel symptom alleviation (63% × 28%) and greater patient satisfaction in the transanal group. However, more functional morbidity was observed with 13% versus 3% of fecal incontinence in the transanal and laparoscopic groups, respectively.

A 2008 Cochrane review analyzed 22 randomized controlled trials of rectocele repair and concluded that posterior vaginal wall repair may be better than transanal repair in the management of rectoceles in terms of recurrence of prolapse.[141]

Table 6 summarizes the results of the different techniques of rectocele repair including their complications.

Stapled transanal rectal resection
STARR was introduced as a surgical option in 1998 when Longo showed his early experience in the treatment of obstructed defecation. Since 1999, the procedure has been performed throughout Europe.[153] In the United States, the experience is still initial, and the clinical pilot study completed the enrollment of patients in 2005. **Fig. 7** illustrates the STARR procedure.

Patients selected for the STARR procedure have prolonged straining, time for evacuation is longer than 10 minutes, they have had sensation of incomplete evacuation for more than 1 year, and there is failure of conservative management. Anorectal physiologic evaluation most commonly reveals rectocele and rectoanal intussusception with normal relaxation of the puborectalis muscle.

Boccasanta and colleagues[153] conducted a prospective multicentric trial enrolling 90 patients. After a 1-year follow-up, 81 patients were satisfied, and only four had poor results. The most common complications observed were 17.8% urgency, 8.9% incontinence to flatus, 5.5% urinary retention, 4.4% bleeding, 3.3% anal stenosis, and 1.1% pneumonia.

Table 6 Results of rectocele repair				
Author	Technique	No of Patients	Success (%)	Follow-up (y)
Hirst et al[142]	TAR	42	48	2
Roman & Michot[143]	TAR	51	50	6
Heriot et al[144]	TAR	45	55	2
Thornton et al[140]	TAR	40	63	3.5
Ayav et al[145]	TAR	21	71	5
Abbas et al[146]	TAR	107	72	4
Tjandra et al[147]	TAR	59	78	1.5
Boccasanta et al[148]	TAR	90	90	—
Van Dam et al[149]	TAR+TV	89	71	2
Yamana et al[150]	TV	30	83	1
De Tayrac et al[151]	TV	25	92.3	2
Rosato[152]	TPR	52	96.2	—

Abbreviations: TAR, Transanal repair; TPR, Transperineal repair; TV, Transvaginal repair.

In 2006, Ommer and colleagues[154] performed STARR in 14 consecutive patients, with good results in all patients after 19 months and a significant decrease in the constipation score. Pechlivanides and colleagues[155] reported their experience with STARR in 16 patients. Improvement of symptoms was noted in only nine. There were no postoperative complications. The seven patients who failed the treatment had documented anismus, and most of them improved after biofeedback. These results show the importance of patient selection before surgical management.

Complications include bleeding from staple line, fecal incontinence, recurrent constipation, and pelvic sepsis.[156–158] A retrospective study conducted by Gagliardi and colleagues[159] including 123 patients who underwent STARR procedure found a 29% incidence of rectocele recurrence and 28% incidence of intussusception recurrence after 17 months. The authors still reported complications, such as postoperative bleeding in 12% and need for reoperation in 19% of the patients.[159,160]

STARR procedure for obstructed defecation related to rectocele and intussusception has promising initial results. Patient selection, and the avoidance of this procedure in patients with documented anismus or paradoxical puborectalis contraction, and proper training can help in avoiding some of the more significant complications.

PUBORECTALIS HYPERTROPHY MANAGEMENT

This is a pathophysiologic entity very similar to paradoxical puborectalis contraction, and its treatment is centered on biofeedback and dietary control. The procedure consists of resection of a V-shaped base of the muscle.

The literature shows different results in terms of solving the constipation problem ranging from less than 10% to 83% in some series.[161–163] Fecal incontinence is a significant concern as well; for these reasons, division of the puborectalis is not commonly recommended.

Sigmoidocele Repair

Sigmoidectomy is the treatment of choice for this cause of obstruction. Limited data have been reported on sigmoidocele treatment. Jorge and colleagues[164] reported

100% success after surgery on grades II and III sigmoidoceles compared with only 33% on patients managed conservatively.

SURGERY FOR SLOW-TRANSIT CONSTIPATION/CI
Colectomy

Patients who have CI with confirmed abnormal transit and normal pelvic floor physiology who do not respond to conservative treatment are candidates for surgery. For over a century, colectomy for constipation has been practiced.[165] Poor success and high complication rates led surgeons to abandon this technique for decades. However, in the past two decades it has returned to practice because of more accurate physiologic studies, which allow a better selection of patients for surgery, as well as the advance in the surgical techniques.

The most widely used technique is the total abdominal colectomy with some anastomotic variations, which include ileorectal, ileosigmoid, or cecorectal. Total abdominal colectomy with ileorectal anastomosis is the treatment of choice for CI, with better results and success rates of more than 90%.[166-169]

A retrospective study examining the long-term follow-up of patients who underwent total abdominal colectomy and ileorectal anastomosis for constipation demonstrated a success rate of 100% with 83% maintaining continence. Only five patients reported one episode of incontinence per month with a mean follow-up of 106 months.[170] The morbidity-mortality of this procedure, however, disincourages its widespread use. The most frequent complication demonstrated is small-bowel obstruction, with an incidence ranging from 7% to 50%.[170-173] Picarsky and colleagues[170] reported a 10% incidence of small-bowel obstruction after 27 months' follow-up. Zutshi and colleagues[174] reported an incidence of 46% of long-term complications in their series, with a 20% incidence of small-bowel obstruction; eight of these patients required re-intervention for lysis of adhesions.

A study by Fan and colleagues[175] from Taiwan showed an improvement in frequency of bowel movements from 1.4 ± 0.9 times per week to 22.8 ± 9 per week after surgery. The incidence of abdominal pain decreased from 75% to 17% of the patients. The two patients who had recurrence of symptoms underwent an ascending rectal anastomosis, which was probably the cause of recurrence. **Table 7** summarizes the results of total abdominal colectomy with ileorectal anastomosis.

Cecorectal anastomosis has the advantage of the absorption of water, sodium, and vitamin B12 and the prevention of renal and gall bladder lithiasis; however, ceacal distension is common with the association of pain and recurrence of constipation.[180] Recently, some authors reported better results using the ceacal reservoir, comparable to ileorectal anastomosis. Iannelli and colleagues[181] completed a prospective follow-up of 14 patients who underwent subtotal colectomy and cecorectal anastomosis and found a significantly increased bowel frequency, ranging from 1.2 ± 0.6/wk to 4.8 ± 7.5/d. Continence was described as perfect by 78.5% of patients, and less than one episode of soiling per week was reported by 14.2%. Postoperative complications occurred in 21.4% of patients with one reoperation; however, there was no mention of long-term complications. Marchesi and colleagues[182] evaluated 43 patients with a mean follow-up of 88.4 months from whom 22 had slow-transit constipation, and 21 had other types of colonic diffuse disease. There were 9.3% of postoperative complications but just one ceacal dilatation with obstructive episodes that required re-operation. Of the slow transit constipation group, all patients had improvement in

Table 7
Results of total abdominal colectomy with Ileorectal anastomosis

Study	No of Patients	Success (%)	Follow-up (mo)
Nylund et al[176]	40	72.5	132
Fitz Harris et al[177]	75	80	—
Fan and Wang[175]	24	82	23
Hassan et al[178]	104	85	104
Webster and Dayton[179]	55	89	12
Zutshi et al[174]	64	92	128
Pikarsky et al[170]	50	100	106

Wexners' constipation score (20.3–2.6), and the quality-of-life index after surgery was close to the mean score for healthy people (115 ± 20).

Sarli and colleagues[183] also had good results with this procedure with a follow-up of 64 months, reporting only one case of constipation easily controlled with laxative. The authors attribute their good results to the selection of the patients, based on careful physiologic assessment and testing. In addition, the type of anastomosis was based on an antiperistaltic anastomosis between the cecum and the rectum, without mesenteric rotation. This is a difference from the original procedure proposed by Deloyers in 1964 and redesigned by Zinzindohué,[183] which involves craniocaudal rotation of the cecum and a consequent torsion of the ileocolic vascular pedicle, causing ischemia and venous stasis. This procedure can lead to intestinal occlusion and cecal distention after surgery. More prospective randomized controlled trials comparing ileorectal anastomosis to cecorectal anastomosis are necessary to prove the safety and efficacy of this anastomosis.

Sigmoid preservation does not have any major technical advantage compared with other procedures and can predispose to postoperative constipation. This is one of the reasons it has not been done.[184] Pemberton and colleagues[184] reported a 50% conversion rate from ileosigmoid anastomosis to ileorectal anastomosis. Sample and colleagues[185] performed 14 laparoscopic subtotal colectomies with ileosigmoid anastomosis. Within 18 months of follow-up, three patients were already requiring laxatives.

Laparoscopic and hand-assisted approaches have increased in the last decade, and for CI they have similar results with faster recovery and cosmetic advantages related to the open technique.[184,185]

Table 8 summarizes the complications and functional results of colectomy for slow-transit constipation.

Segmental colectomy is an alternative that was proposed with the hopes of reducing the risk of side effects of total abdominal colectomy, such as diarrhea and incontinence. However, the results have been poor in terms of treating constipation.[168,188–190] The overall reported success rate was only 68%. Although two studies (1998, 2002) reported good results with 100% success rate and zero degree of incontinence or diarrhea on a follow-up of more than 16 months,[191,192] these results are attributed to a better selection of patients based on the distribution of the markers on the colonic transit study and performance of physiologic tests. However, there is a high incidence of recurrence of constipation, and the surgical morbidity is not as low. For these reasons, segmental colectomy is not the procedure of choice for the majority of surgeons.

Table 8
Complications and bowel frequency after colectomy

Study	No of Patients	Incontinence (%)	Diarrhea (%)	SBO (%)	BM/d (PO)
Fitz Harris et al[177]	75	21	15	16	—
Zutshi et al[174]	64	1.5	7	20	—
Webster and Dayton[179]	55	4	5	8	3
Pikarsky et al[170]	50	17	6	20	2.5
Nylund et al[176]	40	0	—	42.5	3
Thaler et al[186]	17	—	6	—	3.7
Adulaymi et al[187]	15	0	16.7	—	2–6

Abbreviations: BM, bowel movement; PO, by mouth; SBO, small-bowel obstruction.

ANTEGRADE COLONIC ENEMA

Antegrade colonic enema (ACE) was created by Malone[193] in 1990 as a treatment option for patients with severe constipation resistant to conservative methods, where stoma or colectomy would be considered as the only alternatives. It is commonly used by children with neurogenic problems. Some patients with fecal incontinence may benefit from this procedure; however, there is a high incidence of complications. This technique has not gained widespread popularity in North America. The procedure can be performed laparoscopically.

The first description used the reversed appendix as a conduit tunneled into the cecum and to the anterior abdominal wall. This was a modification of the Mitrofanoff procedure, which uses the appendix as a nonrefluxing catheterizable conduit for the bladder. Enemas or irrigation are administered in a distal direction to achieve rectal evacuation.[193]

When the appendix is not available, the cecostomy can be performed using a Chait tube. Modifications of the apendicostomy are usually more complex to create. The ileoceacostomy needs a competent ileoceacal valve to have the continent mechanism. The sigmoid or transverse colon can also be used with an intussuscepted valve constructed from the transected end of the colon.[194,195] Lees and colleagues[196] reported the 36-month follow-up of 32 patients who underwent ACE. Even though the patients had good control of their constipation, they had more than 50% procedure-related complications. The authors also had 59% of conversion of the conduits for other procedures. Stomal stenosis is the most common complication, which is responsible for most of the related procedures or reversion.

In 2007, Altomare and colleagues[197] reported the ACE for 11 patients with severe constipation associated with fecal incontinence, introducing the catheter through the terminal ileum. They showed good results, with quality-of-life improvement and reduction in the Wexner constipation score from 23 to 8.5 However, authors recommend the procedure only as a last option before colostomy.

Sinha and colleagues[198] from UK performed a systematic review of database of 676 patients in 24 studies. Of the procedures, 87% were performed laparoscopically, and the appendix was used in 76% of the cases. The mean volume of enema fluid was 516 mL, and the mean evacuation time was 42 minutes. They found 13% stomal stenosis, which required revision, and social continence was achieved in 93% of the cases. The authors attributed the better results in the last 5 years to with technical advances and an adequate stoma care.

Table 9 summarizes the results of the use of ACE for severe constipation, including some series of children.

This procedure can be an option for palliative treatment and should be considered as an end-stage treatment for severe resistant constipation, such as colostomy or ileostomy.

Ileostomy

STC is rarely treated by ileostomy, because the majority of the patients will not accept a stoma as a definitive treatment. Sometimes, it can be used for patients who have failed after colonic resection. There are a few studies in the literature describing ileostomy for the treatment of constipation, but most of the patients failed previous resections.[202,203]

SNS FOR CONSTIPATION

The affects of SNS on chronic constipation were also observed in patients with simultaneous urinary incontinence.[204] There are only a few reports of SNS for chronic constipation until the present time.[96,112,114,205,206] SNS has been used for several forms of constipation. Ganio and colleagues[207] reported benefits in patients with difficulty in rectal emptying and incomplete evacuation, independent of bowel frequency. However, Kenefick and colleagues[206] included patients with slow bowel frequency and straining. The results of these studies suggest application of SNS and improvement of symptoms for these two different types of constipation.

Ganio and colleagues[114] in 2001 first reported the short-term clinical and physiologic effects of SNS in 10 patients. The authors found significant reduction in difficulty of evacuation, number of unsuccessful visits to the toilet, and in the time necessary to evacuate. All these improvements disappeared after the electrode's removal. At the manometric evaluation, there were increases in amplitude of maximum squeeze pressure and a reduction in the rectal volume for the urge threshold, with a consequent increase in rectal sensation. Malouf and colleagues[205] in the same year also reported the short-term effects of SNS for constipation in 8 patients. Only two patients had improvement in symptoms, and colonic transit did not normalize in any patient. In 2002, the same group published the results of 4 patients with resistant idiopathic constipation. Significant improvement was observed in all patients with temporary implant and in three patients with permanent implant. After 8 months of follow-up, there was improvement in the frequency of bowel movement (6 to 6-28/ 3 wk), median of evacuation score (four versus one), time with bloating (100% versus 12%), time with

Table 9
Results of ACE for constipation

Author	Place of ACE	No of Patients	Follow-up (mo)	Continence (%)	Complications (%)
Kurzcock et al[199]	Colon	8	28	100	50
Altomare et al[197]	Ileum	11	44	—	0
Kim et al[200]	Left colon	19	23	73.7	31
Lees et al[196]	Appendix (54%)	32	36	47	88
King et al[201]	Appendix	42	48	83	42 (infection)
Sinha et al[198]	Appendix (73%)	48	—	92	—

abdominal pain (98% versus 12%), Wexner constipation score (21 versus 9), and quality of life.[208]

Furthermore, Holzer and colleagues[209] studied 19 patients with severe constipation who had positive test stimulation period (100%) and implanted the permanent stimulator. The median stimulation amplitude was 1.5 V. They experienced 42% success after 11 months, with an improvement in the Wexner constipation score, from a baseline of 23 to a median of eight.

Part of the mechanism of action has already been demonstrated in incontinent patients and works for chronic constipation. With the objective of analyzing the effect of SNS on colonic pressure and evaluation of its therapeutic potential, Dinning and colleagues[210] evaluated eight patients with STC, locating a manometric catheter in the colon. The electrical stimulation to S3 increased the pan-colonic antegrade propagating sequence, increasing patient's bowel frequency with a reduction in laxative usage. Some mechanisms of action of SNS were described before. The concern for a significant placebo effect with this expensive method has been addressed. Kenefick and colleagues[211] turned the pulse generator off 1 year after SNS implantation, noticing that all the symptoms returned to baseline rapidly. Holzer and colleagues[209] also reported this effect in one patient who had the electrode disconnected accidentally.

Ganio and colleagues[207] observed some adverse effects of permanent implants in three patients: one infection led to removal and reimplantation, the second patient had recurrent cystitis, and the third had pain at the generator site. Kenefick[208] described only displacement of the device after trauma. Malouf and colleagues[205] did not have any complication but only used the temporary stimulator. Holzer and colleagues[209] did not describe any complications after permanent placement or in the follow-up.

Holzer and colleagues[209] and Kenefick and colleagues[208] addressed quality of life by the 36-item short-form questionnaire and showed improvement in both studies for physical and mental health.

SNS for chronic constipation is a relatively new procedure experience and requires larger prospective comparative studies to prove the true benefit. As with fecal incontinence, the success of SNS is associated with a good selection of patients and positive test stimulation. The results of SNS for constipation are described in **Table 10**.

SNS is a promising option of treatment for fecal incontinent or constipated patients with low morbidity and satisfactory improvement of symptoms. The experience for constipation is initial, but good results for the responder patients have been achieved.

Table 10 Results of SNS for constipation				
Author	No of Patients	Follow-up (mo)	Success (%)	Wexner Constipation Score (B/F)
Malouf et al, 2002[205]	4	8	75	21/9
Ganio et al, 2003[207]	16	12	94.8	14.3/2.7
Kenefick, 2006[208]	4	8	75	21.5/9.2
Holzer et al, 2008[209]	19	11	42	23/8

Abbreviation: B/F-baseline/follow-up.

SUMMARY

Constipation is a very common complaint, often multifactorial in nature. Most patients do not require surgical interventions. Treatment of outlet obstruction is imperative before considering subtotal colectomy for CI. SNS has had some early promising results for both outlet obstruction and CI. The true mechanism of action is unclear.

REFERENCES

1. Madoff RD, Williams JG, Caushaj PE. Fecal incontinence. N Engl J Med 1992; 326:1002–7.
2. Perry S, Shaw C, McGrother C, et al. Prevalence of fecal incontinence in adults aged 40 years or more living in the community. Gut 2002;50:480–4.
3. Roberts RO, Jacobsen SJ, Reilly WT, et al. Prevalence of combined fecal and urinary incontinence: a community-based study. J Am Geriatr Soc 1999;47: 837–41.
4. Browning GG, Parks AG. Postanal repair for neuropathic fecal incontinence: correlation of clinical result and anal canal pressures. Br J Surg 1983;70: 101–4.
5. Jorge JM, Wexner SD. Etiology and management of fecal incontinence. Dis Colon Rectum 1993;36:77–97.
6. Rockwood TH. Incontinence severity and QOL scales for fecal incontinence. Gastroenterology 2004;126:S106–13.
7. Khubchandani IT, Reed JF. Sequelae of internal sphincterotomy for chronic fissure in ano. Br J Surg 1989;76:431–4.
8. Varma A, Gunn J, Gardiner A, et al. Obstetric anal sphincter injury: prospective evaluation of incidence. Dis Colon Rectum 1999;42:1537–43.
9. Rieger N, Schloithe A, Saccone G, et al. A prospective study of anal sphincter injury due to childbirth. Scand J Gastroenterol 1998;33:950–5.
10. Fang DT, Nivatvongs S, Vermeulen FD, et al. Overlapping sphincteroplasty for acquired anal incontinence. Dis Colon Rectum 1984;27:720–2.
11. Parks AG, McPartlin JF. Late repair of injuries of the anal sphincter. Proc R Soc Med 1971;64:1187–9.
12. Tan JJY, Chan M, Tjandra JJ. Evolving therapy for fecal incontinence. Dis Colon Rectum 2007;50:1950–67.
13. Madoff RD, Parker SC, Varma MG, et al. Fecal incontinence in adults. Lancet 2004;364:621–32.
14. Rao SS. Diagnosis and management of fecal incontinence. Am J Gastroenterol 2004;99:1585–604.
15. Muller C, Belyaev O, Deska T, et al. Fecal incontinence: an up-to-date critical overview of surgical treatments options. Langenbecks Arch Surg 2005;390: 544–52.
16. Cook TA, Mortensen NJ. Management of fecal incontinence following obstetric injury. Br J Surg 1998;85:293–9.
17. Elton C, Stoodley BJ. Anterior anal sphincter repair: results in a district general hospital. Ann R Coll Surg Engl 2002;84:321–4.
18. Engel AF, Kamm MA, Sulton AH, et al. Anterior anal sphincter repair in patients with obstetric trauma. Br J Surg 1994;81:1231–4.
19. Oliveira L, Pfeifer J, Wexner SD. Physiological and clinical outcome of anterior sphincteroplasty. Br J Surg 1996;83:502–5.
20. Osterberg A, Edebol K, Graf W. Results of surgical treatment for fecal incontinence. Br J Surg 2000;87:1546–52.

21. Pinta T, Kylänpää-Bäck ML, Salmi T, et al. Delayed sphincter repair for obstetric ruptures. Colorectal Dis 2003;5:73–8.
22. Noderval S, Oian P, Revhaug A, et al. Anal incontinence after obstetric sphincter tears: outcome of anatomic primary repairs. Dis Colon Rectum 2005;48: 1055–61.
23. Malouf AJ, Norton CS, Engel AF, et al. Long-term results of overlapping anterior anal sphincter repair for obstetric trauma. Lancet 2000;355:260–6.
24. Rothbarth J, Bemelman WA, Meijerink WJ, et al. Long-term results of anterior anal sphincter repair for fecal incontinence due to obstetric injury. Dig Surg 2000;17:390–4.
25. Morren GL, Hallbook O, Nystrong PO, et al. Audit of anal-sphincter repair. Colorectal Dis 2001;3:17–22.
26. Grey BR, Sheldon RR, Telford KJ, et al. Anterior anal sphincter repair can be of long-term benefit: a 12-year case cohort from a single surgeon. BMC Surg 2007; 7(1):1–6.
27. Halverson AL, Hull TL. Long-term outcome of overlapping anal sphincter repair. Dis Colon Rectum 2002;45:345–8.
28. Zorcolo L, Covotta L, Bartolo DC. Outcome of anterior sphincter repair for obstetric injury: comparison of early and late results. Dis Colon Rectum 2005; 48:524–31.
29. Barisic GI, Krivokapic ZV, Markovic VA, et al. Outcome of overlapping anal sphincter repair after three months and after a mean of eighty months. Int J Colorectal Dis 2006;21:52–6.
30. Maslekar S, Gardiner AB, Duthie GS. Anterior anal sphincter repair for fecal incontinence: good long-term results are possible. Am Col Surg 2007;204: 40–6.
31. Gutierrez A, Madoff RD, Lowry AC, et al. Long-term results of anterior sphincteroplasty. Dis Colon Rectum 2004;47:727–31.
32. Tjandra JJ, Han WR, Goh J, et al. Direct repair vs. overlapping sphincter repair: a randomized controlled trial. Dis Colon Rectum 2003;46:937–42.
33. Hasegawa H, Yoshioka K, Keighley MR. Randomized trial of fecal diversion for sphincter repair. Dis Colon Rectum 2000;43:961–4.
34. Giordano P, Renzi A, Efron J, et al. Previous sphincter repair does not affect the outcome of repeat repair. Dis Colon Rectum 2002;45:635–40.
35. Pinedo G, Vaizey CJ, Nichols RJ, et al. Results of repeat anal sphincter repair. Br J Surg 1999;86:66–9.
36. Vaizey CJ, Norton C, Thornton MJ, et al. Long-term results of repeat anal sphincter repair. Dis Colon Rectum 2004;47:858–63.
37. Parks AG. Anorectal incontinence. Proc R Soc Med 1975;68:681–90.
38. Abbas SM, Bissett IP, Neill ME, et al. Long-term outcome of post anal repair in the treatment of fecal incontinence. ANZ J Surg 2005;75:783–6.
39. Matsuoka H, Mavrantonis C, Wexner SD, et al. Postanal repair for fecal incontinence: is it worthwhile? Dis Colon Rectum 2000;43:1561–7.
40. Yoshioka K, Keighley MR. Critical assessment of quality of continence after postanal repair for fecal incontinence. Br J Surg 1989;76:1054–7.
41. Bartolo DCC, Roe AM, Locke-Edmunds JC, et al. Flap valve theory of anorectal continence. Br J Surg 1986;73:1012–4.
42. Miller R, Orrom WJ, Cornes H. Anterior sphincter plication and levatorplasty in the treatment of fecal incontinence. Br J Surg 1989;76:1058–60.
43. Dmochowski RR, Appell RA. Injectable agents in the treatment of stress urinary incontinence in women: where are we now? Urologiia 2000;56(6 Suppl 1):32–40.

44. Shafik A. Polytetrafluoroethylene injection for the treatment of partial fecal incontinence. Int Surg 1993;78(2):159–61.
45. Stojkovic SG, Lim M, Burke D, et al. Intra-anal collagen injection for the treatment of faecal incontinence. Br J Surg 2006;93(12):1514–8.
46. Tjandra JJ, Lim JF, Hiscock R, et al. Injectable silicone biomaterial for fecal incontinence caused by internal anal sphincter dysfunction is effective. Dis Colon Rectum 2004;47(12):2138–46.
47. Maeda Y, Vaizey CJ, Kamm MA. Pilot study of two new injectable bulking agents for the treatment of faecal incontinence. Colorectal Dis 2008;10(3):268–72.
48. Van der Hagen SJ, van Gemert WG, Baeten CG. PTQ Implants in the treatment of faecal soiling. Br J Surg 2007;94(2):222–3.
49. Pickrell KL, Broadbent TR, Masters FW, et al. Construction of a rectal sphincter and restoration of anal continence by transplanting the gracilis muscle. Ann Surg 1952;135:853–62.
50. Baeten C, Spaans F, Fluks A. An implanted neuromuscular stimulator for fecal continence following previously implanted gracilis muscle: report of a case. Dis Colon Rectum 1988;31:134–7.
51. Chapman AE, Geerdes B, Hewett P, et al. Systematic review of dynamic graciloplasty in the treatment of fecal incontinence. Br J Surg 2002;89:138–53.
52. Baeten CG, Geerdes BP, Adang EM, et al. Anal dynamic graciloplasty in the treatment of intractable fecal incontinence. N Engl J Med 1995;332:1600–5.
53. Matzel KE, Madoff RD, LaFontaine LJ, et al. Complications of dynamic graciloplasty: incidence, management, and impact on outcome. Dynamic Graciloplasty Therapy Study Group. Dis Colon Rectum 2001;44(10):1427–35.
54. Gurusamy KS, Marzouk D, Benziger H. A review of contemporary surgical alternatives to permanent colostomy. Int J Surg 2005;3(3):193–205. Epub 2005 Sep 21.
55. Madoff RD, Rosen HR, Baeten CG, et al. Safety and efficacy of dynamic muscle plasty for anal incontinence: lessons from a prospective, multicenter trial. Gastroenterology 1999;116(3):549–56.
56. Baeten CG, Bailey HR, Bakka A, et al. Safety and efficacy of dynamic graciloplasty for fecal incontinence: report of a prospective, multicenter trial. Dynamic Graciloplasty Therapy Study Group. Dis Colon Rectum 2000;43(6):743–51.
57. Baeten CG, Uludag OO, Rongen MJ. Dynamic graciloplasty for fecal incontinence. Microsurgery 2001;21(6):230–4.
58. Wexner SD, Baeten C, Bailey R, et al. Long-term efficacy of dynamic graciloplasty for fecal incontinence. Dis Colon Rectum 2002;45(6):809–18.
59. Rongen MJ, Uludag O, El Naggar K, et al. Long-term follow-up of dynamic graciloplasty for fecal incontinence. Dis Colon Rectum 2003;46(6):716–21.
60. Koch SM, Uludağ O, Rongen MJ, et al. Dynamic graciloplasty in patients born with an anorectal malformation. Dis Colon Rectum 2004;47(10):1711–9.
61. Thornton MJ, Kennedy ML, Lubowski DZ, et al. Long-term follow-up of dynamic graciloplasty for faecal incontinence. Colorectal Dis 2004;6(6):470–6.
62. Penninckx F. Belgian experience with dynamic graciloplasty for faecal incontinence. Br J Surg 2004;91(7):872–8.
63. Tillin T, Gannon K, Feldman RA, et al. Third-party prospective evaluation of patient outcomes after dynamic graciloplasty. Br J Surg 2006;93(11):1402–10.
64. Scott FB, Bredley WE, Timm GW. Treatment of urinary incontinence by implantable prosthetic sphincter. Urologiia 1973;1:252–9.
65. Christiansen J, Lorentzen M. Implantation of artificial sphincter for anal incontinence. Lancet 1987;2:244–5.

66. Baxter NN, Rothenberger DA, Lowry AC. Measuring fecal incontinence. Dis Colon Rectum 2003;46:1591–605.
67. Sangwan YP, Coller JA, Barrett RC, et al. Unilateral pudendal neuropathy. Significance and implications. Dis Colon Rectum 1996;39:249–51.
68. Michot F, Tuech JJ, Lefebure B, et al. A new implantation procedure of artificial sphincter for anal incontinence: the transvaginal approach. Dis Colon Rectum 2007;50(9):1401–4.
69. Wong WD, Congliosi SM, Spencer MP, et al. The safety and efficacy of the artificial bowel sphincter for fecal incontinence: results from a multicenter cohort study. Dis Colon Rectum 2002;45:1139–53.
70. Christiansen J, Rasmussen OO, Lindorff-Larsen K. Long-term results of artificial anal sphincter implantation for severe anal incontinence. Ann Surg 1999;230(1):45–8.
71. Lehur PA, Roig JV, Duinslaeger M. Artificial anal sphincter: prospective clinical and manometric evaluation. Dis Colon Rectum 2000;43(8):1100–6.
72. Altomare DF, Dodi G, La Torre F, et al. Multicentre retrospective analysis of the outcome of artificial anal sphincter implantation for severe faecal incontinence. Br J Surg 2001;88(11):1481–6.
73. Ortiz H, Armendariz P, DeMiguel M, et al. Complications and functional outcome following artificial anal sphincter implantation. Br J Surg 2002;89(7):877–81.
74. Devesa JM, Rey A, Hervas PL, et al. Artificial anal sphincter: complications and functional results of a large personal series. Dis Colon Rectum 2002;45(9):1154–63.
75. Michot F, Costaglioli B, Leroi AM, et al. Artificial anal sphincter in severe fecal incontinence: outcome of prospective experience with 37 patients in one institution. Ann Surg 2003;237(1):52–6.
76. Parker SC, Spencer MP, Madoff RD, et al. Artificial bowel sphincter: long-term experience at a single institution. Dis Colon Rectum 2003;46(6):722–9.
77. da Silva GM, Jorge JM, Belin B, et al. New surgical options for fecal incontinence in patients with imperforate anus. Dis Colon Rectum 2004;47(2):204–9.
78. Casal E, San Ildefonso A, Carracedo R, et al. Artificial bowel sphincter in severe anal incontinence. Colorectal Dis 2004;6(3):180–4.
79. La Torre F, Masoni L, Montori J, et al. The surgical treatment of fecal incontinence with artificial anal sphincter implant. Preliminary clinical report. Hepatogastroenterology 2004;51(59):1358–61.
80. O'Brien PE, Dixon JB, Skinner S, et al. A prospective, randomized, controlled clinical trial of placement of the artificial bowel sphincter (Acticon Neosphincter) for the control of fecal incontinence. Dis Colon Rectum 2004;47(11):1852–60.
81. Melenhorst J, Koch SM, van Gemert WG, et al. The artificial bowel sphincter for faecal incontinence: a single centre study. Int J Colorectal Dis 2008;23(1):107–11.
82. Tanagho EA, Schmidt RA. Bladder pacemaker: scientific basis and clinical future. J Urol 1982;20:614–9.
83. Matzel KE, Stadelmaier U, Hohenfellner M, et al. Electrical stimulation for the treatment of fecal incontinence. Lancet 1995;346:1124–7.
84. Ganio E, Realis Luc A, Ratto C, et al. Sacral nerve modulation for fecal incontinence functional results and assessment of quality of life. Available at: www.colorep.it; 2003.
85. Jarrett ME, Varma JS, Duthie GS, et al. Sacral nerve stimulation for fecal incontinence in the UK. Br J Surg 2004;91:755–61.
86. Kenefick NJ, Vaizey CJ, Nicholls RJ, et al. Sacral nerve stimulation for fecal incontinence due to systemic sclerosis. Gut 2002;51:881–3.

87. Cheetham MA, Kenefick NJ, Kamm MA. Non-surgical treatment of fecal incontinence. Hosp Med 2001;62:538–41.
88. Matzel KE, Stadelmaier U, Bittorf B, et al. Bilateral sacral spinal nerve stimulation for fecal incontinence after low anterior rectum resection. Int J Colorectal Dis 2002;17:430–4.
89. Tjandra JJ, Chan MK, Yeh CH, et al. Sacral nerve stimulation is more effective than optimal medical therapy for severe fecal incontinence: a randomized controlled study. Dis Colon Rectum 2008;51:494–502.
90. Vitton V, Gigout J, Grimaud JC, et al. Sacral nerve stimulation can improve continence in patients with Crohn's disease with internal and external anal sphincter disruption. Dis Colon Rectum 2008;51(6):924–7.
91. Tjandra JJ, Lim JF, Matzel K. Sacral nerve stimulation: an emerging treatment for fecal incontinence. ANZ J Surg 2004;74:1098–106.
92. Kenefick NJ, Vaizey CJ, Cohen RC, et al. Medium-term results of permanent sacral nerve stimulation for fecal incontinence. Br J Surg 2002;89:896–901.
93. Michelsen HB, Christensen P, Krogh K, et al. Sacral nerve stimulation for fecal incontinence alters colorectal transport. Br J Surg 2008;95:779–84.
94. Vaizey CJ, Kamm MA, Roy AJ, et al. Double-blind crossover study of sacral nerve stimulation for fecal incontinence. Dis Colon Rectum 2000;43:298–301.
95. Kenefick NJ, Emmanuel A, Nicholls RJ, et al. Effect of sacral nerve stimulation on autonomic nerve function. Br J Surg 2003;90(10):1256–60.
96. Gladman MA, Scott SM, Chan CL, et al. Rectal hyposensitivity: prevalence and clinical impact in patients with intractable constipation and fecal incontinence. Dis Colon Rectum 2003;46:238–46.
97. Holzer B, Rosen HR, Novi G, et al. Sacral nerve stimulation for neurogenic faecal incontinence. Br J Surg 2007;94(6):749–53.
98. Sheldon R, Kiff ES, Clarke A, et al. Sacral nerve stimulation reduces corticoanal excitability in patients with faecal incontinence. Br J Surg 2005;92(11):1423–31.
99. Ratto C, Grillo E, Parello A, et al. Sacral neuromodulation in treatment of fecal incontinence following anterior resection and chemoradiation for rectal cancer. Dis Colon Rectum 2005;48(5):1027–36.
100. Jarrett ME, Matzel KE, Stösser M, et al. Sacral nerve stimulation for faecal incontinence following a rectosigmoid resection for colorectal cancer. Int J Colorectal Dis 2005;20(5):446–51.
101. Uludağ O, Dejong CH. Sacral neuromodulation in patients with fecal incontinence. Dis Colon Rectum 2002;45:A34–6.
102. Rosen HR, Urbarz C, Holzer B, et al. Sacral nerve stimulation as a treatment for fecal incontinence. Gastroenterology 2001;121:536–41.
103. Jarrett ME, Dudding TC, Nicholls RJ, et al. Sacral nerve stimulation for fecal incontinence related to obstetric anal sphincter damage. Dis Colon Rectum 2008;51(5):531–7. Epub 2008 Feb 27.
104. Hetzer FH, Hahnloser D, Clavien PA, et al. Quality of life and morbidity after permanent sacral nerve stimulation for fecal incontinence. Arch Surg 2007; 142(1):8–13.
105. Matzel KE, Kamm MA, Stösser M, et al. Sacral spinal nerve stimulation for faecal incontinence: multicentre study. Lancet 2004;363(9417):1270–6.
106. Melenhorst J, Koch SM, Uludag O, et al. Sacral neuromodulation in patients with faecal incontinence: results of the first 100 permanent implantations. Colorectal Dis 2007;9(8):725–30.
107. Rasmussen OO, Buntzen S, Sørensen M, et al. Sacral nerve stimulation in fecal incontinence. Dis Colon Rectum 2004;47(7):1158–62 [discussion 1162–3].

108. Uludağ O, Koch SM, van Gemert WG, et al. Sacral neuromodulation in patients with fecal incontinence: a single-center study. Dis Colon Rectum 2004;47(8): 1350–7.
109. Brouwer R.G., Duthie G. Sacral nerve stimulation is effective treatment for fecal incontinence in the presence of a sphincter defect or previous sphincter repair [abstract 70]. In: ASCRS 2008, Boston [oral presentation], p. 129.
110. Altomare D, Ratto C, Ganio E, et al. Sacral nerve stimulation in fecal incontinence: results 5 years after implant [abstract 71]. In: ASCRS 2008, Boston, p. 129.
111. Chan MK, Tjandra JJ. Sacral nerve stimulation for fecal incontinence: external anal sphincter defect vs. intact anal sphincter. Dis Colon Rectum 2008;51(7): 1015–24 [discussion: 1024–5].
112. Jarrett ME, Mowatt G, Glazener CM, et al. Systematic review of sacral nerve stimulation for fecal incontinence and constipation. Br J Surg 2004;91: 1559–69.
113. Leroi AM, Michot F, Grise P, et al. Effect of sacral nerve stimulation in patients with fecal and urinary incontinence. Dis Colon Rectum 2001;44:779–89.
114. Ganio E, Masin A, Ratto C, et al. Short–term sacral nerve stimulation for functional anorectal and urinary disturbances: results in 40 patients: evaluation of a new option for anorectal functional disorders. Dis Colon Rectum 2002;44: 1261–7.
115. Ganio E, Luc AR, Clerico G, et al. Sacral nerve stimulation for treatment of fecal incontinence: a novel approach for intractable fecal incontinence. Dis Colon Rectum 2001;44:619–31.
116. Dudding TC, Parés D, Vaizey CJ, et al. Predictive factors for successful sacral nerve stimulation in the treatment of faecal incontinence: a 10-year cohort analysis. Colorectal Dis 2008;10(3):249–56.
117. Lembo T, Camilleri M. Chronic constipation. N Engl J Med 2003;349:1360–8.
118. Connell AM, Hilton C, Irvine G, et al. Variation of bowel habit in two population samples. Br Med J 1965;5470:1095–9.
119. Drossman DA, Cocazziari E, Talley NJ, et al. Rome II: the functional gastrointestinal disorders: diagnosis, pathophysiology and treatment- a multinational consensus In: Drossman DA, Talley NJ, et al, 2nd edition. McLean (VA): Degnon Associates, 2000:382.
120. Agachan F, Chen T, Pfeifer J, et al. A constipation scoring system to simplify evaluation and management of constipated patients. Dis Colon Rectum 1996; 39:681–5.
121. Karasick S, Karasick D, Karasick SR. Functional disorders of the anus and rectum: findings on defecography. AJR Am J Roentgenol 1993;160:777–82.
122. Bartram C. Dynamic evaluation of the anorectum. Radiol Clin North Am 2003;41: 425–41.
123. Preston DM, Lennard-Jones JE. "Severe chronic constipation of young men: idiopathic slow transit constipation." Gut 1986;27:41.
124. Altomare DF, Portincasa P, Rinaldi M, et al. Slow-transit constipation: a solitary symptom of a systemic gastrointestinal disease. Dis Colon Rectum 1999;42: 231–40.
125. Van der Sijp JR, Kamm MA, Nightingale JM, et al. Disturbed gastric and small bowel transit in severe idiopathic constipation. Dig Dis Sci 1993;38:837–44.
126. Donald A, Baxter JN, Bessent RG, et al. Gastric emptying in patients with constipation following childbirth and due to idiopathic slow transit. Br J Surg 1997; 84:1141–3.

127. Johansson C, Nilsson BY, Holmstrőm B, et al. Association between rectocele and paradoxical sphincter response. Dis Colon Rectum 1992;35:503–9.
128. Rosato GO. Rectocele and perineal hernias. In: Beck DE, Wexner SD, editors. Fundamentals in anorectal surgery. London: WB Saunders; 1998. p. 99–114.
129. Mellgreen A, Anzen B, Nilsson B-Y, et al. Results of rectocele repair. A prospective study. Dis Colon Rectum 1995;38:7–13.
130. Pitchford CA. Rectocele: a cause of anorectal pathologic changes in women. Dis Colon Rectum 1967;10:464–6.
131. Arnold MW, Stewart WRC, Aguilar PS. Rectocele repair: four years' experience. Dis Colon Rectum 1990;33:684–7.
132. Rosato G.O. Rectocele repair. Presented at colorectal disease in 1996: an international exchange of medical and surgical concepts, Fort Lauderdale, Fl, February 15–17.
133. Sarles JC, Arnaud A, Selezneff I, et al. Endorectal repair of rectocele. Int J Colorectal Dis 1989;4:167–71.
134. Sehapayak S. Transrectal repair of rectocele: an extended armamentarium of colorectal surgeons. A report of 355 cases. Dis Colon Rectum 1985;28:422–33.
135. Block IR. Transrectal repair of rectoceles using obliterative sutures. Dis Colon Rectum 1986;29:707–11.
136. Rosato GO, Lumi CM. Surgical treatment of rectocele: colorectal approaches. In: Wexner SD, Duthie GS, editors. Constipation: etiology, evaluation and management. 2nd edition. London: Springer; 2006. p. 177–83.
137. Altomare DF, Rinaldi M, Veglia A, et al. Combined perineal and endorectal repair of rectocele by circular stapler. A novel surgical technique. Dis Colon rectum 2002;45:1549–52.
138. Ho YH, Ang M, Nyam D, et al. Transanal approach to rectocele repair may compromise anal sphincter pressures. Dis Colon Rectum 1988;41:354–8.
139. Sullivan ES, Leaverton GH, Hardwick CE. Transrectal perineal repair: an adjunct to improved function after anorectal surgery. Dis Colon Rectum 1968;11:106–14.
140. Thornton MJ, Lam A, King DW. Laparoscopic or transanal repair of rectocele? A retrospective matched cohort study. Dis Colon Rectum 2005;48:792–8.
141. Maher C, Baessler K, Glazener CM, et al. Surgical management of pelvic organ prolapse in women: a short version Cochrane review. Neurourol Urodyn 2008; 27(1):3–12.
142. Hirst GR, Hughes RJ, Morgan AR, et al. The role of rectocele repair in targeted patients with obstructed defecation. Colorectal Dis 2005;7:159–63.
143. Roman H, Michot F. Long-term outcomes of transanal rectocele repair. Dis Colon Rectum 2005;48:510–7.
144. Heriot AG, Skull A, Kumar D. Functional and physiological outcome following transanal repair of rectocele. Br J Surg 2004;91:1340–4.
145. Ayav A, Bresler L, Brunaud L, et al. Long-term results of transanal repair of rectocele using linear stapler. Dis Colon Rectum 2004;47:889–94.
146. Abbas SM, Bissett IP, Neill ME, et al. Long-term results of the anterior Delorme's operation in the management of symptomatic rectocele. Dis Colon Rectum 2005;48:317–22.
147. Tjandra JJ, Ooi BS, Tang CL, et al. Transanal repair of rectocele corrects obstructed defecation if it is not associated with animus. Dis Colon Rectum 1999;42:1544–50.
148. Boccasanta P, Venturi M, Calabro G, et al. Which surgical approach for rectocele? A multicentric report from Italian coloproctologysts. Tech Coloproctol 2001;5(3):149–56.

149. van Dam JH, Huisman WM, Hop WC, et al. Fecal continence after rectocele repair: a prospective study. Int J Colorectal Dis 2000;15(1):54–7.

150. Yamana T, Takahashi T, Iwadare J. Clinical and physiologic outcomes after transvaginal rectocele repair. Dis Colon Rectum 2006;49(5):661–7.

151. de Tayrac R, Picone O, Chauveaud-Lambling A, et al. A 2-year anatomical and functional assessment of transvaginal rectocele repair using a polypropylene mesh. Int Urogynecol J Pelvic Floor Dysfunct 2006;17(2):100–5 Epub 2005 May 21.

152. Rosato GO. Patologia Del piso pelviano- constipacion cronica cirurgia en el sindrome de obstruccion Del tracto de salida (SOTS)- VI curso internacional de coloproctologia 2005 [Spanish].

153. Boccasanta P, Venturi M, Stuto A, et al. Stapled transanal rectal resection for outlet obstruction: a prospective, multicenter trial. Dis Colon Rectum 2004; 47(8):1285–96 [discussion 1296–7].

154. Ommer A, Albrecht K, Wenger F, et al. Stapled transanal rectal resection (STARR): a new option in the treatment of obstructive defecation syndrome. Langenbecks Arch Surg 2006;391(1):32–7.

155. Pechlivanides G, Tsiaoussis J, Athanasakis E, et al. Stapled transanal rectal resection (STARR) to reverse the anatomic disorders of pelvic floor dyssynergia. World J Surg 2007;31(6):1329–35.

156. Dodi G, Pietroletti R, Milito G, et al. Bleeding, incontinence, pain and constipation after STARR transanal double stapling rectotomy for obstructed defecation. Tech Coloproctol 2003;7(3):148–53.

157. Bassi R, Rademacher J, Savoia A. Rectovaginal fistula after STARR procedure complicated by haematoma of the posterior vaginal wall: report of a case. Tech Coloproctol 2006;10(4):361–3.

158. Pescatori M, Dodi G, Salafia C, et al. Rectovaginal fistula after double-stapled transanal rectotomy (STARR) for obstructed defaecation. Int J Colorectal Dis 2005;20(1):83–5.

159. Gagliardi G, Pescatori M, Altomare DF, et al. Results, outcome predictors, and complications after stapled transanal rectal resection for obstructed defecation. Dis Colon Rectum 2008;51(2):186–95 [discussion: 195]. Epub 2007 Dec 22.

160. Pescatori M, Boffi F, Russo A, et al. Complications and recurrence after excision of rectal internal mucosal prolapse for obstructed defecation. Int J Colorectal Dis 2006;21:160–5.

161. Wasserman JF. Puborectalis syndrome: rectal stenosis due to anorectal spasm. Dis Colon Rectum 1964;7:87–98.

162. Kawano M, Fujioshi T, Takagi K. Puborectalis syndrome. J Jpn Soc Coloproctol 1987;40:612.

163. Barnes PRH, Hawley PR, Preston DM, et al. Experience of posterior division of the puborectalis muscle in the management of chronic constipation. Br J Surg 1985;72:475–7.

164. Jorge JM, Yang Y-K, Wexner SD. Incidence and clinical significance of sigmoidoceles as determined by a new classification system. Dis Colon Rectum 1994; 37:1112–7.

165. Lane WA. Remarks on the results of treatment of chronic constipation. BMJ 1908;1:1126–30.

166. Beck DE, Jagelman DG, Fazio VW. Surgery of idiopathic constipation. Gastroenterol Clin North Am 1987;16:143–56.

167. Vasilevsky CA, Nemer FD, Balcos EG, et al. Is subtotal colectomy a viable option in the management of chronic constipation. Dis Colon Rectum 1988;31: 679–81.

168. Rughes ES, McDermortt FT, Johnson WR, et al. Surgery for constipation. Aust N Z J Surg 1981;51:144–8.
169. Zenilman ME, Dunnegan DL, Sopen NJ, et al. Successful surgical treatment of idiopathic colonic dismotility. The role of prospective evaluation of coloanal motor function. Arch Surg 1999;124:947–51.
170. Pikarsky AJ, Singh JJ, Weiss EG, et al. Long-term follow up of patients undergoing colectomy for colonic inertia. Dis Colon Rectum 2001;4:179–83.
171. Piccirillo MF, Reissman P, Carnavos R, et al. Colectomy as treatment for constipation in selected patients. Br J Surg 1995;82:898–901.
172. Kamm MA, Hawley PR, Lennard-Jones JE. Outcome of colectomy for severe idiopathic constipation. Gut 1988;29:969–73.
173. Gilbert KP, Lewis FG, Billingham RP, et al. Surgical treatment of constipation. West J Med 1984;140:569–72.
174. Zutshi M, Hull TL, Trzcinski R, et al. Surgery for slow transit constipation. Are we helping patients? Int J Colorectal Dis 2007;22:265–9.
175. Fan CW, Wang JY. Subtotal colectomy for colonic inertia. Int Surg 2000;85:309–12.
176. Nylund G, Oresland T, Fasth S, et al. Long-term outcome after colectomy in severe idiopathic constipation. Colorectal Dis 2001;3(4):253–8.
177. FitzHarris GP, Garcia-Aguilar J, Parker SC, et al. Quality of life after subtotal colectomy for slow-transit constipation: both quality and quantity count. Dis Colon Rectum 2003;46(4):433–40.
178. Hassan I, Pemberton JH, Tonia M, et al. Ileorectalanastomosis for slow transit constipation: long-term functional and quality of life results. J Gastrointest Surg 2006;10:1330–7.
179. Webster C, Dayton M. Results after colectomy for colonic inertia: a sixteen-year experience. Am J Surg 2001;182:639–44.
180. Fasth S, Hedlund H, Savaninger G, et al. Functional results after subtotal colectomy and caecorectal anastomosis. Acta Chir Scand 1983;149:623–7.
181. Iannelli A, Fabiani P, Mouiel J, et al. Laparoscopic subtotal colectomy with cecorectal anastomosis for slow-transit constipation. Surg Endosc 2006;20(1):171–3. Epub 2005 Nov 24.
182. Marchesi F, Sarli L, Percalli L, et al. Subtotal colectomy with antiperistaltic cecorectal anastomosis in the treatment of slow-transit constipation: long-term impact on quality of life. World J Surg 2007;31(8):1658–64.
183. Sarli L, Iusco D, Donadei E, et al. The rationale for cecorectal anastomosis for slow transit constipation. Acta Biomed 2003;74(Suppl 2):74–9.
184. Pemberton JH, Rath DM, Ilstrup DM. Evaluation and surgical treatment of severe chronic constipation. Ann Surg 1991;214:403–13.
185. Sample C, Grupta R, Bamebriz F, et al. Laparoscopic subtotal colectomy for colonic inertia. J Gastrointest Surg 2005;9:803–8.
186. Thaler K, Dinnewitzer A, Oberwalder M, et al. Quality of life after colectomy for colonic inertia. Tech Coloproctol 2005;9:133–7.
187. Aldulaymi BH, Rasmussen O, Christiansen J. Long-term results of subtotal colectomy for severe slow-transit constipation in patients with normal rectal function. Colorectal Dis 2001;3(6):392–5.
188. Cirocco WC. Segmental colectomy in the management of colonic inertia. Am Surg 1999;65:901–2.
189. Metcalf AM, Phillips SM, Zinsmeister AR, et al. Simplified assessment of segmental colonic transit. Gastroenterology 1987;92:40–7.
190. Pfeifer J, Agachan F, Wexner SD. Surgery for constipation. A review. Dis Colon Rectum 1996;39:444–60.

191. Lundin E, Karlbom U, Pahlman L, et al. Outcome of segmental colonic resection for slow transit constipation. Br J Surg 2002;89:1270–4.

192. You YT, Wang JY, Changchien CR, et al. Segmental colectomy in the management of colonic inertia. The Am Surg 1998;64:775–7.

193. Malone PS, Ransley PG, Kiely EM. Preliminary report: the antegrade continence enema. Lancet 1990;336:1217–8.

194. Hughes SF, Williams NS. Continent colonic conduit for the treatment of fecal incontinence associated with disordered evacuation. Br J Surg 1995;82:1318–20.

195. Williams NS, Hughes SF, Stuchfield B. Continent colonic conduit for rectal evacuation in severe constipation. Lancet 1994;343:1321–4.

196. Lees NP, Hodson P, Hill J, et al. Long-term results of the antegrade continent enema procedure for constipation in adults. Colorectal Dis 2004;6:362–8.

197. Altomare DF, Rinaldi M, Rubini D, et al. Long-term functional assessment of antegrade colonic enema for combined incontinence and constipation using a modified Marsh and Kiff technique. Dis Colon Rectum 2007;50(7):1023–31.

198. Sinha CK, Grewal A, Ward HC. Antegrade continence enema (ACE): current practice. Pediatr Surg Int 2008;24(6):685–8. Epub 2008 Apr 12.

199. Kurzrock EA, Karpman E, Stone AR. Colonic tubes for the antegrade continence enema: comparison of surgical technique. J Urol 2004;172(2):700–2.

200. Kim SM, Han SW, Choi SH. Left colonic antegrade continence enema: experience gained from 19 cases. J Pediatr Surg 2006;41(10):1750–4.

201. King SK, Sutcliffe JR, Southwell BR, et al. The antegrade continence enema successfully treats idiopathic slow-transit constipation. J Pediatr Surg 2005;40(12):1935–40.

202. Scarpa M, Barollo M, Keighley RB. Ileostomy for constipation. Long-term post operative outcome. Colorectal Dis 2005;7:224–7.

203. El-Tawil AM. Reasons for creation of permanent ileostomy for management of idiopathic chronic constipation. J Gastroenterol Hepatol 2004;19:844–6.

204. Caraballo R, Bologna RA, Lukban J, et al. Sacral nerve stimulation as a treatment for urge incontinence and associated pelvic floor disorders at a pelvic floor center: a follow-up study. Urologiia 2001;57(Suppl 1):121.

205. Malouf AJ, Wiesel PH, Nicholls T, et al. Short-term effects of sacral nerve stimulation for idiopathic slow transit constipation. World J Surg 2002;26:166–70.

206. Kenefick NJ, Nicholls RJ, Cohen RJ, et al. Permanent sacral nerve stimulation for treatment of idiopathic constipation. Br J Surg 2002;89:882–8.

207. Ganio E, Masin A, Ratto C, et al. Sacral nerve modulation for chronic outlet obstruction. Available at: www.colorep.it.

208. Kenefick NJ. Sacral nerve neuromodulation for the treatment of lower bowel motility disorders. Ann R Coll Surg Engl 2006;88(7):617–23.

209. Holzer B, Rosen HR, Novi G, et al. Sacral nerve stimulation in patients with severe constipation. Dis Colon Rectum 2008;51:524–30.

210. Dinning PG, Fuentealba SE, Kennedy ML, et al. Sacral nerve stimulation induces pan-colonic propagating pressure waves and increases defecation frequency in patients with slow-transit constipation. Colorectal Dis 2007;9(2):123–32.

211. Kenefick NJ, Vaizey CJ, Cohen CR, et al. Double-blind placebo-controlled crossover study of sacral nerve stimulation for idiopathic constipation. Br J Surg 2002;89(12):1570–1.

Constipation: Evaluation and Treatment of Colonic and Anorectal Motility Disorders

Satish S.C. Rao, MD, PhD, FRCP (Lon)[a,b,*]

KEYWORDS

- Constipation • Irritable bowel syndrome • Colon
- Dyssynergic defecation • Anorectal manometry
- Balloon expulsion test

Constipation is a polysymptomatic disorder and not a single disease. Because it represents many symptoms that affect colonic and anorectal function, the estimates of its prevalence have been imprecise. Likewise, the number of patients with this condition who seek medical care and the costs of diagnostic tests or treatment are not accurately known. This article focuses on the colonic and anorectal motility disturbances that are associated with chronic constipation and their management.

EPIDEMIOLOGY

Recent estimates based on householder surveys in North America suggest a prevalence rate of 15% to 20% for chronic constipation.[1–3] However, other figures have been quoted and the discrepancies in the literature are largely due to how the problem has been defined or reported. The prevalence of constipation increases with age, especially in those over the age of 65 years.[4–6] It also affects work-related productivity and leads to more absences from school.[7] Constipation is associated with significantly lower quality of life and higher psychological distress.[8] Furthermore, these

This article appeared previously in the September 2007 issue of Gastroenterology Clinics of North America (36:3), with permission.

This work was supported in part by grant DK57100-0441 from the National Institutes of Health and in part by the Department of Internal Medicine, University of Iowa Carver College of Medicine.

[a] Division of Gastroenterology & Hepatology, Department of Internal Medicine, University of Iowa Carver College of Medicine, Iowa City, IA, USA

[b] Division of Gastroenterology, University of Iowa Hospitals and Clinics, 200 Hawkins Drive, 4612 JCP, Iowa City, IA-52242, USA

* Division of Gastroenterology, University of Iowa Hospitals and Clinics, 200 Hawkins Drive, 4612 JCP, Iowa City, IA-52242.

E-mail address: satish-rao@uiowa.edu

Gastrointest Endoscopy Clin N Am 19 (2009) 117–139
doi:10.1016/j.giec.2008.12.006
1052-5157/08/$ – see front matter © 2009 Elsevier Inc. All rights reserved.

effects tend to be more common in patients with constipation-predominant irritable bowel syndrome (IBS-C) and dyssynergia than in patients with slow transit constipation.[9,10] A recent community survey estimated an average cost of $200 per patient within a large health maintenance organization group for the management of constipation.[11]

FUNCTIONAL SUBTYPES

There is emerging consensus amongst experts that in the absence of alarm symptoms, such as weight loss, bleeding, recent change in bowel habit, and significant abdominal pain; or secondary causes, such as drugs, metabolic disorders, colorectal cancer, or local painful lesions, such as anal fissure,[12] most patients with a complaint of constipation have a functional disorder affecting the colon or anorectum. At least three subtypes have been recognized, although overlap exists. Slow transit constipation is characterized by prolonged delay in the transit of stool through the colon. This delay may be due to a primary dysfunction of the colonic smooth muscle (myopathy) or its nerve innervation (neuropathy), or it could be secondary to an evacuation disorder, such as dyssynergic defecation. Dyssynergic defecation, also known as obstructive defecation,[13] anismus,[14] pelvic floor dyssynergia,[15] or outlet obstruction,[16,17] is characterized by either difficulty or inability with expelling stool from the anorectum.[13] Many patients with dyssynergic defecation also have prolonged colonic transit.[9] A third subtype is comprised of patients with IBS-C in whom abdominal pain, with or without bloating, is a prominent symptom together with altered bowel habit.[18] These subjects may or may not have slow transit or dyssynergia.

DEFINITION

Recent reviews and guidelines have addressed issues related to the definition of this common complaint.[15,19–23] Although infrequent defecation has generally been used to define constipation, such symptoms as excessive straining, passage of hard stools, or feeling of incomplete evacuation have only recently been recognized as equally important and perhaps more common.[1] Thus, a definition that does not address the heterogeneity of symptoms that affect a patient with constipation is not only inaccurate, but also may lead to inadequate management.

To improve the diagnosis of constipation and to develop more uniform standards for performing clinical research, consensus criteria have been proposed by an international panel of experts.[13,21,23,24] Rome III criteria define functional constipation primarily on the basis of symptoms alone,[23,24] whereas dyssynergic defecation is defined both on the basis of symptoms and objective physiological criteria.[13,25] The Rome III criteria for functional constipation.[24] is shown in **Box 1**.[26] A modification of the Rome III criteria[23] for dyssynergia is shown in **Box 2**.

PATHOPHYSIOLOGY

The right colon performs several complex functions that include mixing, fermentation and salvage of the ileal effluent, secretion, and desiccation of the intraluminal contents to form stool. The left colon serves as a conduit for desiccation and more rapid transport of stool and the rectosigmoid region serves as a sensorimotor organ that facilitates the awareness, retention, and evacuation of stool when socially conducive. These functions are regulated by neurotransmitters, such as serotonin, acetylcholine, calcitonin gene-related peptide and substance P; intrinsic colonic reflexes; and

---

Box 1

Diagnostic criteria for functional constipation with criteria fulfilled for the last 3 months and symptom onset at least 6 months before diagnosis

1. Must include two or more of the following:

   a. Straining during at least 25% of defecations

   b. Lumpy or hard stools in at least 25% of defecations

   c. Sensation of incomplete evacuation following at least 25% of defecations

   d. Sensation of anorectal obstruction or blockage during at least 25% of defecations

   e. Manual maneuvers to facilitate for at least 25% of defecations (eg, digital evacuation, support of the pelvic floor)

   f. Fewer than three defecations per week

2. Loose stools rarely present without the use of laxatives

3. Insufficient criteria for IBS

From Longstreth GF, Thompson WG, Chey WD, et al. Functional bowel disorders. Gastroenterology 2006;130:1480–91; with permission.

---

a plethora of learned and reflex mechanisms that govern stool transport and evacuation, most of which are incompletely understood.

Constipation may result from structural, mechanical, metabolic, or functional disorders that affect the colon or anorectum either directly or indirectly. As demonstrated in a study of healthy subjects showing that defecation could be postponed for several days,[27] there is a significant interaction between the brain and the gut. This means that neurological dysfunction and abnormalities of afferent and efferent brain–gut connections may have profound effects on colonic and anorectal function.

Pathophysiology of Slow Transit Constipation

Because colonic motor activity is intermittent, variable, and influenced by sleep, waking, meals,[28–30] physical[31] and emotional stressors,[32–34] and differences in regional colonic motor function,[35] the pathophysiology of constipation continues to evolve.

Box 2

Criteria for dyssynergic defecation

A. Patients must fulfill the symptomatic criteria for functional constipation as defined in **Box 1**.

B. Constipated patients must fulfill two or more of the following physiologic criteria:

   1. Dyssynergic pattern of defecation (types 1–3; see **Fig. 3**)

   2. Inability to expel a balloon or stool-like device, such as a fecom, within 1 minute.

   3. A prolonged colonic transit time (ie, >6 markers on a plain abdominal radiograph taken 120 hours after ingestion of one Sitzmarks capsule containing 24 radio-opaque markers)

   4. Inability to expel barium or >50% retention during defecography

From Rao SSC. Dyssynergic defecation. Gastroenterol Clin North Am 2001;30:97–114; with permission.

However, recent studies have shed more light. It has been shown that patients with slow transit constipation exhibit significant impairment of phasic colonic motor activity both in stationary[28] and in prolonged 24-hour ambulatory colonic motility recordings.[36,37] Furthermore, it has been shown that the gastrocolonic responses following a meal (**Fig. 1**) and the morning waking responses after sleep are also significantly diminished, but the diurnal variation of colonic motor activity is preserved.[37] In contrast, periodic rectal motor activity, a three-cycles-per-minute activity that predominately occurs in the rectum and rectosigmoid region and is invariably seen at nighttime,[38] significantly increases in patients with slow transit constipation.[39] This excessive uninhibited distal colonic activity may serve as a nocturnal break and retard colonic propulsion of stool.[39] Previous studies have shown that the high amplitude, prolonged duration, propagated contractions (HAPCs) are significantly decreased in constipated

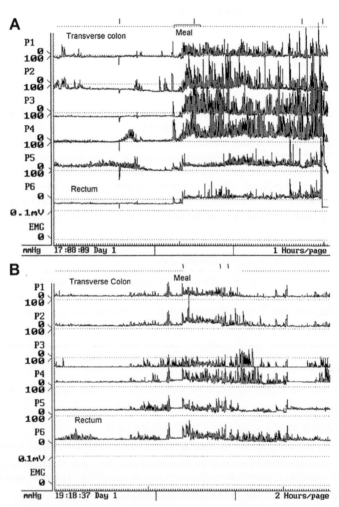

Fig. 1. The effects of a meal on a six-channel colonic manometry recording in a normal subject (*A*) and in a patient with slow transit constipation (*B*). Constipated patients show impaired postprandial or gastrocolonic motor response.

patients.[40,41] Furthermore, in constipated patients, the velocity of propagation is slower, waves have a greater tendency to abort prematurely, and their amplitude is also decreased.[40,42]

Studies that have combined manometry with barostat recordings have shown decreased colonic tone and phasic responses to a meal, although the barostat measurements per se could not distinguish patients with normal transit, slow transit, or pelvic floor dysfunction.[19,43,44] Slow transit constipation may also be associated with autonomic dysfunction.[45,46] Several recent studies have demonstrated a paucity of interstitial cells of Cajal, suggesting the possibility of an underlying neuropathy in these individuals.[47] Because these observations were made on colectomy specimens obtained from patients with chronic constipation, it is unclear whether they represent a primary entity or whether they are secondary to the use of drugs, the use of cathartics, or behavioral changes over many years. Rarely, slow transit constipation may be associated with a more generalized dysmotility and forms part of a pseudo-obstruction syndrome.[48,49]

Because constipation is associated with hard stools, one possible hypothesis is that excessive absorption of water from stool may desiccate colonic contents. However, the colonic absorptive function seems to be relatively well preserved in patients with constipation.[50] In one study, abnormally impaired hormonal responses to ingested water load were reported, but its significance is unclear.[51] Finally, in younger adults, more women than men seek medical help for constipation, suggesting a possible role for endocrine or hormonal imbalance.[51] A decreased level of ovarian and adrenal steroid hormones has been reported,[52] but has not been confirmed. In fact, routine estrogen and progesterone levels are not impaired in most women with constipation. Also, the relationship between menstrual cycle and gut transit remains controversial.[52] Both slower transit during the luteal phase[53] and normal transit have been reported.[54] Studies of neurotransmitters in the colonic wall have also provided conflicting data.[55] A decrease in vasoactive intestinal polypeptide levels[56] and an increase in serotonin levels in the circular muscle[57] have been reported. In an intriguing study of G-protein–mediated smooth muscle contractility, colectomy specimens from women with slow transit constipation showed down-regulation of progesterone-dependent contractile G proteins and up-regulation of inhibitory G proteins when compared with those from nonconstipated controls.[58] These changes were probably due to an over-expression of progesterone receptors.[59] This study offers some mechanistic insights as to why women are more prone to constipation. Most recently, it has been observed that there is a higher prevalence of methanogenic flora in constipated patients[60–62] and that infusion of methane gas impairs muscle contractions.[63] Further study is needed to determine whether methanogenic flora predisposes an individual to develop constipation or is a consequence of altered colonic physiology.

Pathophysiology of Dyssynergic Defecation

In two thirds of patients, dyssynergic defecation appears to be an acquired behavioral disorder of defecation. In the remaining one third, the process of defecation may not have been learnt in childhood.[9] Earlier studies suggested that paradoxical anal contraction or involuntary anal spasm (anismus) during defecation might cause dyssynergic defecation.[14,17,64] Of healthy subjects, 20% to 30% may also exhibit paradoxical anal contraction.[35,65,66] Based on the notion that dyssynergic defecation is a spasmodic dysfunction of the anal sphincter, myectomy of the anal sphincter has been performed.[17,67] Although preliminary studies were encouraging, a more critical assessment has shown that myectomy helps only 10% to 30% of patients.[67] Similarly, most patients who received botulinum toxin injections as a method of paralyzing the anal sphincter muscle and reversing the anal spasm did not improve.[68,69]

In a prospective study, most patients with dyssynergic defecation showed abnormal coordination of the abdominal, rectoanal, and pelvic floor muscles during attempted defecation.[25] This failure of rectoanal coordination may consist of several mechanisms that include impaired rectal contraction, paradoxical anal contraction, or inadequate anal relaxation.[25] Thus, incoordination or dyssynergia of the muscles involved in defecation is most likely responsible for this problem.[13] Additionally, nearly half of dyssynergic patients exhibited impaired rectal sensation.[25]

CLINICAL FEATURES

Constipated patients present with a constellation of symptoms that include a feeling of incomplete evacuation; excessive straining; passage of hard, pellet-like stool; digital disimpaction or vaginal splinting; a lump-like sensation; or blockage in the anal region.[9,13] Additionally, they may report infrequent defecation, often less than three bowel movements per week; abdominal or anorectal discomfort; pain; or bloating.[9] Patients may misrepresent their symptoms or may feel embarrassed to admit the use of digital maneuvers to disimpact stool or to splint their vagina to facilitate defecation. However, by establishing a trustworthy relationship or through the use of symptom questionnaires or stool diaries,[9] it is possible to define the nature of bowel dysfunction in these patients.

A detailed inquiry that includes the nature of the problem, precipitating events, the duration and severity of the problem, and its onset, whether from childhood or following surgery, may all prove beneficial. A long history of recurring problems refractory to dietary measures or laxatives often suggest a functional colorectal disorder, whereas a history of recent onset should alert the physician to seek and exclude an organic illness, including neoplastic disease. The history should also include an assessment of stool frequency, stool consistency, stool size, and degree of straining during defecation, and a history of ignoring a call to stool. The Bristol Stool Scale is an invaluable tool in the assessment of constipation. This not only correlates with transit time but is also the best descriptor of stool form and consistency.[70,71] A dietary history should include an assessment of the amount of fiber and fluid intake, the number of meals, and when they are consumed. Many patients tend to skip breakfast as a result of the "early morning rush." This may prove to be a handicap because there is a two- to threefold increase in colonic motility after waking[30] and after a meal.[28,29] Thus, skipping breakfast and not devoting time toward bowel function in the morning may deprive the colon of an important physiological stimulus. The history should also include the number and type of laxatives and frequency of their use. A family history of using laxatives and a family history of bowel dysfunction may also be important. In one survey, a family history was noted in 30% of patients.[9] Obstetrical, surgical, and drug history is also useful. A history of back trauma or neurological problems may provide additional clues regarding the etiology of constipation. In the elderly, fecal incontinence may be a presenting symptom of stool impaction. However, symptoms alone do not appear to differentiate constipated patients into the three common pathophysiologic subgroups.[72]

In a prospective survey of 120 patients with dyssynergic defecation, excessive straining was reported by 85% of patients, a feeling of incomplete evacuation by 75%, the passage of hard stools by 65%, and a stool frequency of fewer than three bowel movements per week by 62%.[9] Amongst this group, 66% used digital maneuvers to facilitate defecation.[9] In another study of 134 patients, two or fewer stools per week, laxative dependency, and constipation since childhood were associated with slow transit constipation, whereas backache, heartburn, anorectal surgery, and a lower prevalence of normal stool frequency were reported by patients with pelvic floor dysfunction.[73] It was concluded from this study that symptoms were good predictors of transit time, but poor predictors of pelvic floor dysfunction. In another study of 190 patients, stool frequency alone was of little value in the evaluation of constipation but a sense of obstruction or digital-assisted evacuation was specific but not sensitive for difficult defecation.[72] Thus, symptom assessment should be combined with objective testing to better assess the nature of a patient's complaint.

PHYSICAL EXAMINATION

A thorough physical examination that includes a detailed neurological examination should be performed to exclude systemic illnesses that may cause constipation. The abdomen must be carefully examined for the presence of stool, particularly in the left or right lower quadrant. A normal physical examination is not uncommon but it is important to exclude a gastrointestinal mass. Anorectal inspection may reveal skin excoriation, skin tags, anal fissure, or hemorrhoids. Perineal sensation and the anocutaneous reflex can be assessed by gently stroking the perineal skin in all four quadrants with the help of a cotton bud (Q-Tip) or with a blunt needle. Normally, stroking the perianal skin invokes a reflex contraction of the external anal sphincter. If absent, one should clinically suspect neuropathy.

A careful digital rectal examination should be performed to identify the presence of a rectal stricture, stool, or blood in the stool. During digital examination, it is important to ask the patient to bear down as if to defecate. During this maneuver, the examiner should perceive relaxation of the external anal sphincter together with perineal descent. If these features are absent, one should suspect functional obstructive or dyssynergic defecation.[13]

DIAGNOSTIC PROCEDURES

The first step in making a diagnosis of constipation is to exclude an underlying metabolic or pathologic disorder because constipation may be the first symptom of many organic conditions, such as colon cancer. A complete blood count, biochemical profile, serum calcium, glucose levels, and thyroid function tests are usually sufficient for screening purposes. If there is a high index of suspicion, serum protein electrophoresis, urine porphyrins, serum parathyroid hormone, and serum cortisol levels may be requested. Most patients, once organic disorders have been excluded, are found to have a functional neuromuscular disorder. An evaluation of the distal colonic mucosa through flexible sigmoidoscopy may provide evidence for chronic laxative use or may reveal melanosis coli or other mucosal lesions, such as solitary ulcer syndrome, inflammation, or malignancy. Slow transit constipation may coexist with dyssynergic defecation [25,74] and hence assessment of colonic transit together with anorectal function is useful.

RADIOGRAPHIC STUDIES

A plain radiograph of the abdomen may provide evidence for an excessive amount of stool in the colon. If colonoscopy has not been performed, a barium enema may be useful for excluding colonic pathology. Patients with constipation may have a redundant sigmoid colon, a megacolon, or megarectum. The presence of Hirschsprung's disease can also be detected by barium enema, although manometry and histology are required to confirm the diagnosis.

Colonic Transit Study

Because a patient's recall of stool habit is often inaccurate, an assessment of colonic transit time enables the physician to better understand the rate of stool movement through the colon.[75] Several techniques have been described for performing this test.[29] These include the single capsule technique[4] and the multiple capsule technique.[76] The validity of multiple capsule techniques has been questioned.[77] However, for routine clinical purposes, a single capsule technique is sufficient. This test is performed by having the patient swallow a single Sitzmarks capsule (Konsyl Pharmaceuticals, Fort Worth, Texas) containing 24 radio-opaque markers on day 1 and by obtaining a plain radiograph of the abdomen on day 6 (ie, 120 hours later). This study may reveal one of three patterns:

Normal transit: less than five markers remaining in the colon.[19]
Slow transit: six or more markers scattered throughout the colon
Functional obstructive or dyssynergic defecation pattern: six or more markers in the rectosigmoid region with a near normal transit of markers through the rest of the colon

Two thirds of patients with dyssynergic defecation may exhibit a mixed pattern consisting of both slow transit and obstructive delay.[25] In some patients with constipation, the colon transit time may be normal. In these subjects it is important to exclude pelvic floor dysfunction.

Assessment of colonic transit using a novel, wireless capsule technique—SmartPill (SmartPill Corporation, Buffalo, New York)—provides a noninvasive technique of assessing not only colonic transit time but also simultaneously gastric emptying and small bowel transit time (**Fig. 2**). It also provides information regarding colonic contractile

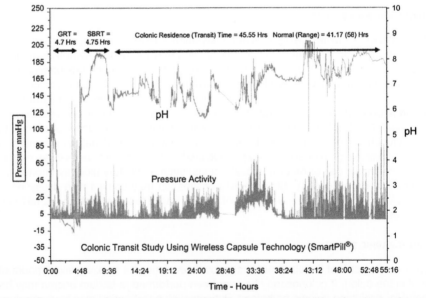

Fig. 2. Whole gut transit time in a patient with slow transit constipation showing prolonged colonic residence time as assessed by wireless capsule technology (SmartPill). The gastric and small bowel residence times appear to be within normal limits. GRT, gastric residence time; SBRT, small bowel residence time.

activity and pH. Preliminary studies in healthy controls have shown that the colonic transit time as assessed by the SmartPill correlates very well with that of the Sitzmarks technique.[78]

Anorectal Manometry

Anorectal manometry provides a comprehensive assessment of the pressure activity in the rectum and anal sphincter region together with an assessment of rectal sensation, rectoanal reflexes, and rectal compliance.[34,35] The technique of anorectal manometry and its utility has been discussed previously.[35] It helps to exclude the possibility of Hirschsprung's disease. Normally, when a balloon is distended in the rectum, there is reflex relaxation of the internal anal sphincter that is mediated by the myenteric plexus. This reflex response is absent in patients with Hirschsprung's disease, but this condition is rare in adults.

Manometry helps to detect abnormalities during attempted defecation. When a subject attempts to defecate normally, rectal pressure rises. This rise is synchronized with a fall in anal sphincter pressure, in large part due to relaxation of the external anal sphincter (**Fig. 3**). This maneuver is under voluntary control and is primarily a learned response. The inability to perform this coordinated movement represents the chief pathophysiologic abnormality in patients with dyssynergic defecation.[13,25] This inability may be due to impaired rectal contraction, paradoxical anal contraction, impaired anal relaxation, or a combination of these mechanisms. Based on these features, at least three types of dysfunction have been recognized:[79]

Type 1: The patient can generate an adequate pushing force (rise in intra-abdominal and intrarectal pressure) along with a paradoxical increase in the anal sphincter pressure.

Type 2: The patient is unable to generate an adequate pushing force (no increase in intrarectal pressure), but can exhibit a paradoxical anal contraction.

Type 3: The patient can generate an adequate pushing force (increase in intrarectal pressure), but has absent or incomplete (<20%) sphincter relaxation (ie, no decrease in anal sphincter pressure).

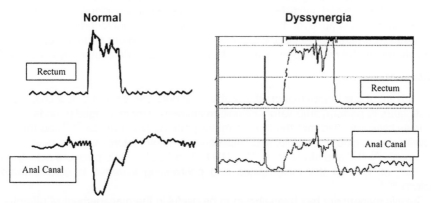

Fig. 3. A normal and abnormal (dyssynergic) pattern of defecation. A normal pattern consists of a rise in the intrarectal pressure coordinated with relaxation of anal sphincter pressure. In contrast, a dyssynergic pattern is associated with a paradoxical increase in anal sphincter pressure. Typical patterns for a normal and dyssynergic pattern of defecation as measured during anorectal manometry with a pressure sensor in the rectum and a pressure sensor in the anal canal.

In addition to the motor abnormalities just described, sensory dysfunction may also be present. The threshold for first sensation and the threshold for a desire to defecate may be higher in about 60% of patients with dyssynergic defecation.[25] This may also be associated with increased rectal compliance. During attempted defecation, some subjects may not produce a normal relaxation largely because of the laboratory conditions.[35,65] Hence, the occurrence of this pattern alone should not be considered as diagnostic of dyssynergic defecation (see diagnostic criteria). By observing the manometric recordings during attempted defecation, it is possible to identify the sequence that most closely resembles a normal pattern of defecation (see **Fig. 3**). This recording can be used to measure the intrarectal pressure, the anal residual pressure, and the percentage of anal relaxation.[35,65] From these measurements, it is possible to estimate an index of the forces required to perform defecation—the defecation index.[35] The defecation index may serve as a simple and quantifiable measure of the recto-anal coordination during defecation.[13,35]

Balloon Expulsion Test

This test provides an assessment of the patient's ability to defecate in the laboratory. Either a silicone-filled stool-like device such as the fecom[80] or a 4-cm long balloon filled with 50 mL of warm water is placed in the rectum.[35] A stopwatch is started and the attendant leaves the room to provide privacy for the patient during balloon expulsion. The patient is asked to expel the device and then immediately stop the clock. Most normal subjects can expel a stool-like device within 1 minute.[35] If the patient is unable to expel the device within 3 minutes, the clinician should suspect dyssynergic defecation.

Defecography

Defecography provides useful information about anatomical and functional changes of the anorectum. It is performed by placing approximately 150 mL of barium into the patient's rectum and having the subject squeeze, cough, and bear down. In patients with dyssynergic defecation, the test may reveal poor activation of levator muscles, prolonged retention of contrast material, inability to expel the barium, or the absence of a stripping wave in the rectum. Patients may find this test embarrassing. Also, the type and consistency of barium paste varies considerably among different centers.[80] Because of these inherent deficiencies, defecography should be regarded as an adjunct to clinical and manometric assessment of anorectal function and should not be relied upon as a sole test for assessing defecatory dysfunction.[23]

Colonic Manometry

The advent of solid-state manometry probes and portable recorders now enables investigators to perform ambulatory colonic manometry over prolonged periods.[29,30,34] Studies have revealed that the colonic motor patterns are complex[34,79] and that the activity is intermittent, variable, and influenced by many factors, such as sleep, waking, meals,[29,30,34] and stressors.[30,33,81] The hallmarks of colonic pressure activity are HAPCs, as well as the meal-related and postwaking increase in colonic motor activity.[34,37]

Colonic manometry has been shown to be useful in the management of refractory constipation in children,[82] but a recent study showed that the test is also useful in adults and can facilitate the selection of patients for surgery.[37] In a case-controlled study, most patients with manometric features of colonic neuropathy (absence of any two of three normal colonic motor responses and presence of HAPCs, gastrocolonic response, and morning waking response) failed to respond to aggressive medical treatment and had a better clinical outcome after colectomy, whereas those with a myopathy and those with a normal colonic motor activity responded adequately to medical treatment.[37] Thus, colonic manometry can serve as an adjunct to current methods of assessing colonic function, particularly in patients with severe constipation.[37] An evidence-based summary of the utility of physiologic and imaging tests in the evaluation of chronic constipation[83] is shown in **Table 1**.[84]

MANAGEMENT OF CONSTIPATION

The first step in managing constipation is to exclude a secondary cause for constipation. This can be accomplished by performing the appropriate tests outlined above. Constipation may be caused by anatomical lesions of the colon or rectum, endocrine or metabolic disorders, neurologic diseases, or a variety of drugs.[12] Constipation is a common and often overlooked adverse effect of many drugs. Some drugs have anticholinergic effects, others desiccate stool, and several others, including analgesics, can cause constipation by altering colonic motility, by interfering with intrinsic colonic reflexes, or by reducing the awareness for stooling. A few other factors merit further discussion. An evidence-based summary of treatment options for chronic constipation[85,86] is shown in **Table 2**.

Fluid Intake and Exercise

General measures that include adequate hydration, regular nonstrenuous exercise, and dedicated time for passing bowel movements may all be useful, but there is little evidence to support this. In a small study (six tests and nine controls) of healthy volunteers, consumption of extra fluid produced no difference in stool output.[87] The role of exercise in improving colonic function is also controversial. Epidemiologic studies suggest that sedentary folks are three times more likely to report constipation.[88] However, the effects of exercise and gut transit time are inconsistent. A recent study showed that exercise decreases the number of phasic contractions in the colon and that this effect depends on the intensity of exercise.[31] Also, there was a proportionate increase in the number of propagated contractions, particularly in the postexercise period, which may accelerate colonic transit.[31]

Most patients who have a normal bowel pattern usually empty stools at approximately the same time every day.[89] This fact suggests that the initiation of defecation is in part a conditioned reflex. Therefore, ritualizing bowel habit may be useful and it is advisable to encourage patients to establish a regular pattern of bowel movement. Colonic motor activity is more active after waking and after a meal.[29,30] Hence, the optimal time for bowel movement is usually within the first 2 hours after waking and after breakfast. Other general measures include timed toilet training that consists of educating patients to attempt a bowel movement at least twice a day, usually 30 minutes after meals, and to strain for no more than 5 minutes. During attempted defecation, patients must be instructed to push at a level of 5 to 7, assuming a maximum effort of straining of 10. They should also be encouraged to capitalize on the physiological events that stimulate colonic motility, such as the waking and the postprandial gastrocolonic responses.[13]

Diet and Fiber

A high fiber diet increases stool weight and accelerates colonic transit time.[90] In contrast, diet that is deficient of fiber may lead to constipation.[90,91] Constipated patients who had either slow transit or pelvic floor dysfunction responded poorly to dietary supplementation with 30 g of fiber per day, whereas those patients without an underlying

Table 1
Evidence-based summary of the utility of physiologic tests for chronic constipation

| Test | Clinical Utility | | | Evidence | Recommendation (Grade)[a] | Comment |
	Strength	Weakness				
Colonic transit study with radio-opaque markers	Evaluates presence of slow, normal, or rapid colonic transit; inexpensive and widely available	Inconsistent methodology; validity has been questioned		Good	B2	Useful to classify patients according to pathopysiological subtypes
Colonic transit study with scintigraphy	Evaluates presence of slow, normal, or rapid colonic transit; provides a whole evaluation of the gut transit	Expensive, time-consuming, limited availability, lack of standardization		Good	B2	Useful to classify patients according to pathopysiological subtypes
Anorectal manometry	Identifies dyssynergic defecation, rectal hyposensitivity, rectal hypersensitivity, impaired compliance, Hirschsprung's disease	Lack of standardization		Good	B2	Useful to establish the diagnoses of Hirschsprung's disease, dyssynergic defecation, and rectal hypo- and hypersensitivity
Balloon expulsion test	Simple, inexpensive, bedside assessment of the ability to expel a simulated stool; identifies dyssynergic defecation	Lack of standardization		Good	B2	Normal balloon expulsion test does not exclude dyssynergia; should be interpreted alongside results of other anorectal tests
Colonic manometry	Identifies colonic myopathy, neuropathy, or normal function facilitating selection of patients for surgery	Invasive, not widely available, lack of standardization		Fair	B3	Adjunct to colorectal function tests; useful before considering colectomy

Grade A1: excellent evidence in favor of the test based on high specificity, sensitivity, accuracy, and positive predicative values. Grade B2: good evidence in favor of the test with some evidence on specificity, sensitivity, accuracy, and predictive values. Grade B3: fair evidence in favor of the test with some evidence on specificity, sensitivity, accuracy, and predictive values. Grade C: poor evidence in favor of the test with some evidence on specificity, sensitivity, accuracy, and predictive values.
[a] *Grades for levels of evidence modified from* Sackett DL. Rules of evidence and clinical recommendations on the use of antithrombotic agents. Chest 1986;89:2S–3S.
Modified from Remes-Troche JM, Rao SS. Diagnostic testing in patients with chronic constipation. Curr Gastroenterol Rep 2006;8:422.

Table 2
Evidence-based summary for the treatment of constipation

Treatment Modalities Commonly Used for Constipation	Recommendation Level and Grade of Evidence
Bulking agents	
• Psyllium	Level II; grade B
• Calcium polycarbophil	Level III; grade C
• Bran	Level III; grade C
• Methycellulose	Level III; grade C
Osmotic laxatives	
• Lactulose	Level II; grade B
• Polyethylene glycol	Level I; grade A
Wetting agents	
• Dioctyl sulfosuccinate	Level III; grade C
Stimulant laxatives	
• Senna	Level III; grade C
• Bisacodyl	Level III; grade C
Others	
• Tegaserod	Level I; grade A
• Lubiprostone	Level I; grade B
Biofeedback therapy for dyssynergic defecation	Level I; grade A
Surgery in the treatment of severe colonic inertia	Level II; grade B

Level I: good evidence—consistent results from well-designed, well-conducted studies. Level II: fair evidence—results show benefit, but strength is limited by the number, quality, or consistency of the individual studies. Level III: poor evidence—insufficient because of limited number or power of studies, and flaws in their design or conduct. Grade A: good evidence in support of the use of a modality in the treatment of constipation. Grade B: moderate evidence in support of the use of a modality in the treatment of constipation. Grade C: poor evidence to support a recommendation for or against the use of the modality. Grade D: moderate evidence against the use of the modality. Grade E: good evidence to support a recommendation against the use of a modality.
Data from Remes-Troche JM, Rao SSC. Defecation disorders: neuromuscular aspects and treatment. Curr Gastroenterol Rep 2006;8(4):291–9.

motility disorder either improved or became symptom-free.[92] Thus, fiber intake may not be a panacea for all patients. A systematic review found 18 double-blind studies related to this issue.[93] Six trials that evaluated bulk laxatives or dietary fiber showed an average weighted increase of 1.4 (95% CI, 0.6–2.2) bowel movements per week, whereas the seven trials that evaluated laxative agents other than bulk, showed an increase of 1.5 (95% CI, 1.1–1.8) bowel movements per week. Other direct comparisons between laxatives and fiber were inconclusive because of the limited number of studies, small sample size, and problems with methodology. With regards to symptom improvement, fiber consistently decreased abdominal pain and improved stool consistency, but the difference was not statistically significant when compared with other laxatives.[93] In general, a fiber intake of 20 to 30 g of fiber per day is optimal.

Laxatives

Laxatives still remain the mainstay of treatment for constipation. About $821 million was spent on over-the-counter laxatives in the United States.[94] Several recent reviews have discussed the common classification of laxatives, their mode of action, the recommended dosage, and potential side effects.[19,20] In addition, a meta-analysis has examined the use of bulk and nonbulk laxatives in patients with constipation.[93] Although there are a variety of preparations, including several over-the-counter compounds, the laxatives that are frequently recommended include milk of magnesia, lactulose, senna compounds, bisacodyl, and polyethylene glycol preparations. In a trial of constipated elderly patients, sorbitol administered as 70% syrup was as efficacious as lactulose in improving symptoms but was cheaper and better tolerated during a 4-week trial.[95] In another trial of 77 elderly nursing home residents, a senna fiber combination was felt to be better than lactulose in improving stool frequency, stool consistency, and ease of passage. In terms of costs, the senna fiber combination was 40% cheaper.[96]

Polyethylene glycol is a large polymer that is not degraded by bacteria and serves as an osmotic laxative. Recent double-blind studies conducted over a 2-week[97] and an 8-week period[98] showed that polyethylene glycol 3350 solutions increased stool frequency and improved bowel symptoms. In a long-term multicenter study of polyethylene glycol 4000, 14.6 g twice a day improved stool frequency, reduced straining effort, softened stools, and decreased the need for oral laxatives and enemas compared with placebo.[99] Among those who completed the study, the stool frequency at baseline was 1.5 versus 1.8; after 2 weeks of treatment with polyethylene glycol 4000 was 8.3 versus 7.4; and after 6 months of polyethylene glycol or placebo was 7.7 versus 5.4, respectively. Thus, polyethylene glycol may be effective in the long term. However, there was a 30% dropout in the polyethylene glycol group and a 60% dropout in the placebo group, raising concerns about efficacy and tolerance. Hence, confirmatory trials are awaited.

Slow Transit Constipation

Before labeling a patient as suffering with either slow transit constipation or colonic inertia, it is important to exclude pelvic floor dysfunction. Ideally, slow transit constipation should be treated with an agent that restores normal colonic function. **Table 2**[86] shows a list of agents that are currently available or in phase III/IV clinical trials for the treatment of constipation. These include secretagogues and prokinetics. Drugs in the former category include lubiprostone, colchicine, and misoprostol.[100]

Lubiprostone is an oral bicyclic fatty acid that belongs to a new class of drugs called prostones. It activates the type 2 chloride channels that are located on the intestinal epithelial cell leading to an active secretion of chloride in the intestinal lumen.[101] In healthy humans, a whole-gut scintigraphic study reported that lubiprostone slowed gastric emptying, but accelerated small bowel transit time and colonic transit time at 24 hours.[102] In randomized controlled studies with an intention to treat analysis, lubiprostone significantly increased the number of spontaneous bowel movements per week, improved straining effort, raised overall satisfaction with bowel habit, and produced softer stools when compared with placebo.[103]

Likewise, recent studies of tegaserod, which is a serotonin compound and a 5-hydroxytryptamine 4 ($5HT_4$) partial agonist, revealed that the drug accelerates gastric emptying and colonic transit time.[104] Furthermore large randomized controlled trails in United States and Europe have revealed that tegaserod increases the number of complete spontaneous bowel movements per week, relieves other bothersome constipation-related symptoms, and improves overall bowel satisfaction.[103,105] Recent open-labeled studies reveal that the effects of the drug are sustained over 12 months. Just recently, sales of tegaserod have been suspended because of a 0.01% incidence of coronary and cerebrovascular events. Hence, the drug is not currently available.

Table 3 provides information regarding the drug profiles for lubiprostone and tegaserod.

Emerging Therapies

A number of treatments are currently being investigated in clinical trials. Renzapride and mosapride are both 5-hydroxytryptamine 3 ($5\text{-}HT_3$) agonists–$5\text{-}HT_4$ antagonists that have very similar mechanisms of action. In preliminary studies, both agents demonstrated clinically significant dose-related acceleration of colonic transit. Currently, renzapride is being evaluated in IBS-C patients and there is also potential to research the effects of the agents in patients with chronic constipation.[106] Another drug, alvimopan, is a peripherally acting μ–opioid receptor antagonist. This agent does not cross the blood–brain barrier and, therefore, does not inhibit the analgesic effect of opioids. In a physiologic study, alvimopan reversed opioid-induced delayed colonic transit in healthy subjects.[107] Another 21-day randomized trial assessed alvimopan in 168 patients with opioid-induced bowel dysfunction. Within 8 hours of treatment, at least one bowel movement was achieved in 54% of subjects who received 1 mg alvimopan and in 43% of those who received 0.5 mg compared with 29% of those who received placebo.[108] Alvimopan is effective in the treatment of acute postoperative ileus.[109] Linaclotide, a guanylate cyclase C agonist accelerates gut transit and is being tested in patients with constipation.[110,111]

Dyssynergic Defecation

The treatment of a patient with dyssynergic defecation consists of standard treatment for constipation, including diet, laxatives, timed toilet training, and other measures outlined above, together with specific treatment consisting of neuromuscular conditioning using biofeedback techniques.[13] Other avenues that have been tried include botulinum toxin injection,[68,69] anal myectomy, and surgical approaches.[17,67] Details regarding the specifics of performing biofeedback therapy have been discussed previously.[13] The purpose of biofeedback therapy is to restore a normal pattern of defecation by using an instrument-based education program. The primary goals are

Table 3
Pharmacologic profiles of lubiprostone and tegaserod

	Lubiprostone	Tegaserod
Drug class	Chloride channel activator	$5HT_4$ agonist
Mechanism of action	Increases intestinal fluid secretion	Stimulates the peristaltic reflex
		Stimulates intestinal secretion
		Inhibits visceral sensitivity
Indications	Chronic idiopathic constipation in male and female patients	Chronic idiopathic constipation in male and female patients aged <65 years, IBS-C in female patients
Dose and administration	24 μg twice daily orally with food	6 mg twice daily orally before meals
Adverse events	Nausea (31.1%)	Headache (15%)
	Diarrhea (13.2%)	Diarrhea (7%)
	Headache (13.2%)	Abdominal pain (5%)
	Abdominal pain (6.7%)	Nausea (5%)

to correct the underlying dyssynergia that affects the abdominal, rectal, and anal sphincter muscles, and to improve the rectal sensory perception.

Patients are initially taught diaphragmatic breathing techniques to improve their abdominal pushing effort and to synchronize this with anal relaxation. Thereafter, visual or auditory feedback techniques are used to provide input to the patient regarding his or her performance during attempted defecation maneuvers. The patient's posture and breathing techniques are also corrected using verbal reinforcement techniques. The number of training sessions should be customized to the patient's need.

Three recent randomized controlled studies have bolstered the evidence supporting the use of biofeedback therapy in dyssynergic defecation. Chiarioni and colleagues[112] compared polyethylene glycol (n = 55) with five weekly biofeedback sessions (n = 54) in patients who were nonresponders to conservative therapy. At 6 months, major improvements were reported by patients enrolled in the biofeedback arm (43 of 54 or 80%) compared with the polyethylene glycol and counseling group (12 of 55 or 22%). The benefit of biofeedback was sustained at 12 and 24 months. A second study by Chiarioni[113] in 2005 compared the benefits of biofeedback in patients with slow transit constipation to those with dyssynergia. At 6 months, greater improvement was seen in the dyssynergia group compared with the slow transit only group (71% versus 8% reported improved satisfaction). This study suggests that biofeedback helps patients with dyssynergia but not patients with slow transit. Finally, a recent study by Rao and colleagues[114] compared biofeedback with sham biofeedback or standard therapy of diet, exercise, and laxatives in 77 patients. Dyssynergia was corrected in 79% of patients in the biofeedback group compared with 4% in the sham group. The number of complete spontaneous bowel movements was higher in the biofeedback group compared with sham group (**Fig. 4**), and overall bowel satisfaction also improved in the biofeedback group. Balloon expulsion time and the colonic transit time decreased significantly in the biofeedback group. Thus, biofeedback therapy appears to be the preferred method of treatment for patients with dyssynergic defecation.

Stool Impaction and Refractory Constipation Including Surgery

Patients with stool impaction or those with hard stools that are difficult to expel require digital disimpaction. This can be painful and may require sedation or anesthesia. Once

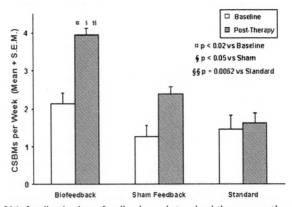

Fig. 4. Effects of biofeedback, sham feedback, and standard therapy on the number of complete spontaneous bowel movements per week in patients with dyssynergic defecation. (*From* Rao SS, Seaton K, et al. Randomized controlled trial of biofeedback, sham feedback, and standard therapy for dyssynergic defecation. Clin Gastroenterol Hepatol 2007;5:335; with permission.)

the colon has been cleaned, these patients require a rigorous bowel-conditioning regime of laxatives and suppositories to prevent stool impaction. Glycerin or bisacodyl suppository together with enemas are usually successful, but have not been prospectively assessed. Additional measures include saline or osmotic laxatives or polyethylene glycol solutions. After establishing a bowel regime, it is important to assess these patients for an underlying colonic or generalized motility disorder.

In patients with constipation that is refractory to medical therapy, surgery can be an option. However, before considering surgery, it is important to establish that the problem is confined to the colon and does not represent a generalized neuromuscular dysfunction of the gut. It has been suggested that segmental colonic resection may be beneficial in some situations, particularly in children.[115] Controlled data are lacking however. Children with refractory constipation may also have neuromuscular dysfunction confined to well-defined colonic segments.[115] Surgical options for refractory constipation include colectomy and ileostomy or ileorectal anastomosis.[116] The use of laparoscopic colectomy may further help to improve this procedure.[117] In a large series of carefully selected patients, results of surgery were quite favorable.[116] However, surgery should be considered as a last resort for patients with constipation. It is important to emphasize that colectomy with ileorectal anastomosis does not improve symptoms in patients with dyssynergic defecation unless their dyssynergia has been corrected. Similarly, colectomy may not offer symptom relief for constipated patients with abdominal pain or psychosocial problems.[118]

EVIDENCE-BASED SUMMARY FOR THE TREATMENT OF CONSTIPATION

A systematic review of the literature using an evidence-based approach for various treatment options is summarized in **Table 2**. For each specific content area, the supporting evidence was graded using a three-point graded scale.[86] Level 1 evidence was derived from one or more randomized clinical trials. Level 2 evidence was supported by one or more well-designed cohort or case-control studies. Level 3 evidence was derived from expert opinion, based on clinical experience. Evidence was further subdivided into five categories: A—good evidence in favor of the intervention; B—moderate evidence in favor of the intervention; C—poor evidence to support a recommendation for or against the use of the intervention; D—moderate evidence against the intervention; E—good evidence against the intervention.

SUMMARY

Constipation is a common polysymptomatic clinical disorder that affects up to 20% of the world's population. It leads to significant economic burden, loss of work-related productivity, and diminished quality of life. Studies over the past decade have led to an improved understanding of the underlying mechanisms, especially as they relate to colonic and anorectal function. Although many conditions, such as metabolic problems, fiber deficiency, anorectal problems, and drugs, can cause constipation, when these conditions are excluded, functional chronic constipation consists of three overlapping subtypes: slow transit constipation, dyssynergic defecation, and irritable bowel syndrome with constipation. The Rome criteria may serve as a useful guide for making a clinical diagnosis of functional constipation. Today, an evidence-based approach can be used to treat patients with chronic constipation. The availability of specific drugs for the treatment of chronic constipation, such as tegaserod and lubiprostone, has enhanced the therapeutic armamentarium for the management of these patients. Randomized controlled trials have also established the efficacy of biofeedback therapy in the treatment of dyssynergic defecation.

REFERENCES

1. Pare P, Ferrazzi S, Thompson WG, et al. An epidemiological survey of constipation in canada: definitions, rates, demographics, and predictors of health care seeking. Am J Gastroenterol 2001;96:3130–7.
2. Stewart WF, Liberman JN, Sandler RS, et al. Epidemiology of constipation (EPOC) study in the United States: relation of clinical subtypes to sociodemographic features. Am J Gastroenterol 1999;94:3530–40.
3. Pare P, Ferrazzi S, Thompson WG. A Longitudinal Survey of Self-reported Bowel Habits in the United States. Dig Dis Sci 1989;34:1153–62.
4. Talley NJ, Fleming KC, Evans JM, et al. Constipation in an elderly community: a study of prevalence and potential risk factors. Am J Gastroenterol 1996;91: 19–25.
5. Sonnenberg A, Koch TR. Physician visits in the United States for constipation: 1958 to 1986. Dig Dis Sci 1989;34:606–11.
6. Higgins PD, Johanson JF. Epidemiology of constipation in North America: a systematic review. Am J Gastroenterol 2004;99:750–9.
7. Martin BC, Barghout V, Cerulli A. Direct medical costs of constipation in the United States. Manag Care Interface 2006;19:43–9.
8. Chang L, Toner BB, Fukudo S, et al. Gender, age, society, culture, and the patient's perspective in the functional gastrointestinal disorders. Gastroenterology 2006;130:1435–46.
9. Rao SS, Tuteja AK, Vellema T, et al. Dyssynergic defecation: demographics, symptoms, stool patterns, and quality of life. J Clin Gastroenterol 2004;38: 680–5.
10. Pare P, Gray J, Lam S, et al. Health-related quality of life, work productivity, and health care resource utilization of subjects with irritable bowel syndrome: baseline results from LOGIC (Longitudinal Outcomes Study of Gastrointestinal Symptoms in Canada), a naturalistic study. Clin Ther 2006;28:1726–35, discussion 1710–1.
11. Singh G. Use of Health Care Resources and Cost of Care for Adults With Constipation. Clin Gastroenterol Hepatol 2007 Jul 9 [Epub ahead of print].
12. Rao SSC. Constipation-Method of Conn's Current Therapy. In: Rakel RE, editor. Philadelphia: W.B. Saunders Company; 1999. p. 20–3.
13. Rao SSC. Dyssynergic Defecation. Gastroenterol Clin North Am. Volume 30 2001;97–114.
14. Preston DM, Lennard-Jones JE. Anismus in Chronic Constipation. Dig Dis Sci 1985;30:413–8.
15. Whitehead WE, Devroede G, Habib FI, et al. Functional Disorders of the Anorectum. Gastroenterology International 1992;5:92–108.
16. Kawimbe BM, Papachrysostomou M, Binnie NR, et al. Outlet Obstruction Constipation (Anismus) Managed by Biofeedback. Gut 1991;32:1175–9.
17. Martelli H, Devroede G, Arhan P, et al. Mechanisms of Idiopathic Constipation: Outlet obstruction. Gastroenterology 1978;75:623–31.
18. Mertz H, Naliboff B, Mayer E. Physiology of Refractory Chronic Constipation. Am J Gastroenterol 1999;94:609–15.
19. Bharucha AE, Phillips SF. Slow Transit Constipation. Gastroenterol Clin North Am 2001;30:77–95.
20. Locke GR 3rd, Pemberton JH, Phillips SF. American Gastroenterological Association Medical Position Statement: guidelines on constipation. Gastroenterology 2000;119:1761–6.

21. Thompson WG, Longstreth GF, Drossman DA, et al. Functional Bowel Disorders and Functional Abdominal Pain. Gut 1999;45:1143–7.
22. Whitehead WE, Devrode G, Habib F, et al. Functional Disorders of the Anus and Rectum. In: Drossman DA, editor. The Functional Gastrointestinal Disorders. Boston: Little Brown & Company; 1994. p. 217–63.
23. Whitehead WE, Wald A, Diamant NE, et al. Functional disorders of the anus and rectum. Gut 1999;45(Suppl. 2):II55–9.
24. Bharucha AE, Wald A, Enck P, et al. Functional anorectal disorders. Gastroenterology 2006;130:1510–8.
25. Rao SSC, Welcher KD, Leistikow JS. Obstructive Defecation: A Failure of Rectoanal Coordination. Am J Gastroenterol 1998;93:1042–50.
26. Longstreth GF, Thompson WG, Chey WD, et al. Functional bowel disorders. Gastroenterology 2006;130:1480–91.
27. Klauser AG, Voderholzer WA, Heinrich CA, et al. Behavioural Modification of Colonic Function: Can Constipation be Learned? Dig Dis Sci 1990;35:1271–5.
28. Bassotti G, Betti C, Imbimbo BP, et al. Colonic Motor Response to Eating: A Manometric Investigation in Proximal and Distal Portion of the Viscus in Man. Am J Gastroenterol 1989;84–6.
29. Rao SSC, Kavelock R, Beaty J, et al. Effects of Fat and Carbohydrate Meals on Colonic Motor Response. Gut 2000;46:205–11.
30. Rao SSC, Sadeghi P, Beaty J, et al. Ambulatory 24-h Colonic Manometry in Healthy Humans. Am J Physiol Gastrointest Liver Physiol 2001;280:G629–39.
31. Rao SSC, Beaty J, Chamberlain M, et al. Effects of Acute Graded Exercise on Human Colonic Motility. Am J Physiol 1999;276:G1221–6.
32. Chowdhury AB, Dinoso VP, Lorber SH. Characterization of a Hyperactive Segment at the Rectosigmoid Junction. Gastroenterology 1976;71:584–8.
33. Narducci F. Twenty four hour manometric recordings of colonic motor activity in man. Gut 1987;28:17–25.
34. Rao SS, Patel RS. How useful are manometric tests of anorectal function in the management of defecation disorders? Am J Gastroenterol 1997;92:469–75.
35. Rao SSC, Hatfield R, Soffer E, et al. Manometric Tests of Anorectal Function in Healthy Adults. Am J Gastroenterol 1999;94:773–83.
36. Rao S. Colonic motor patterns in healthy humans: A 24 hour ambulatory study. Gastroenterology 1998;A114–829.
37. Rao SS, Sadeghi P, Beaty J, et al. Ambulatory 24-hour colonic manometry in slow-transit constipation. Am J Gastroenterol 2004;99:2405–16.
38. Rao SSC, Welcher K, Hatfield R. Periodic Rectal Motor Activity (PRMA): The Intrinsic Colonic Gatekeeper. Gastroenterology 1995;108.
39. Rao SS, Sadeghi P, Batterson K, et al. Altered periodic rectal motor activity: a mechanism for slow transit constipation. Neurogastroenterol Motil 2001;13:591–8.
40. Rao SSC, Sadeghi P, Kavlock R, et al. Specialized Propagating Contractions (SPC) in Health and Constipation. Gastroenterology 1999;116:G4635.
41. Bassotti G. Manometric investigation of high amplitude propagated contractile activityof the human colon. Am J Physiology 1988;255:G660–4.
42. Rao SSC, Sadeghi P, Kavlock R, et al. Specialized Propagating Pressure Waves (SSPW) in Health and Constipation. Am J Gastroenterol 1999;94:A2684.
43. Law NM, Bharucha AE, Zinsmeister AR. Rectal and colonic distension elicit viscerovisceral reflexes in humans. Am J Physiol Gastrointest Liver Physiol 2002;283:G384–9.

44. O'Brien MD. Camilleri M, von der Ohe MR, et al. Motility and tone of the left colon in constipation: a role in clinical practice? Am J Gastroenterol 1996;91:2532–8.
45. Knowles CH, Scott M, Lunniss PJ. Outcome of colectomy for slow transit constipation. Ann Surg 1999;230:627–38.
46. Surrenti E, Rath DM, Pemberton JH, et al. Audit of Constipation in a Tertiary Referral Gastroenterology Practice. Am J Gastroenterol 1995;90:1471–5.
47. He CL, Burgart L, Wang L, et al. Decreased interstitial cell of cajal volume in patients with slow-transit constipation. Gastroenterology 2000;118:14–21.
48. Mollen RM, Hopman WP, Kuijpers HH, et al. Abnormalities of upper gut motility in patients with slow-transit constipation. Eur J Gastroenterol Hepatol 1999;11: 701–8.
49. Spiller RC. Upper gut dysmotility in slow-transit constipation: is it evidence for a pan-enteric neurological deficit in severe slow transit constipation? Eur J Gastroenterol Hepatol 1999;11:693–6.
50. Devroede G, Soffie M. Colonic Absorption in Idiopathic Constipation. Gastroenterology 1973;64:552–61.
51. Preston DM, Lennard-Jones J. Severe Chronic Constipation of Young Women: Idiopathic Slow Transit Constipation? Gut 1986;27:41–8.
52. Kamm MA, Farthing MJ, Lennard-Jones JE. Bowel function and transit rate during the menstrual cycle. Gut 1989;30:605–8.
53. Wald A, Van Thiel DH, Hoechstetter L, et al. Gastrointestinal transit: the effect of the menstrual cycle. Gastroenterology 1981;80:1497–500.
54. Turnbull GK, Thompson DG, Day S, et al. Relationships between symptoms, menstrual cycle and orocaecal transit in normal and constipated women. Gut 1989;30:30–4.
55. Kamm MA. Pathophysiology of Constipation. In: Phillips SF, Shorter RG, editors. The Large Intestine. Physiology, Pathophysiology and Disease. New York: Raven Press; 1991. p. 709–26.
56. Koch TR, Carney JA, Go L, et al. Idiopathic chronic constipation is associated with decreased colonic vasoactive intestinal peptide. Gastroenterology 1988; 94:300–10.
57. Lincoln J, Crowe R, Kamm MA, et al. Serotonin and 5-hydroxyindoleacetic acid are increased in the sigmoid colon in severe idiopathic constipation. Gastroenterology 1990;98:1219–25.
58. Xiao ZL, Pricolo V, Biancani P, et al. Role of progesterone signaling in the regulation of G-protein levels in female chronic constipation. Gastroenterology 2005; 128:667–75.
59. Xiao ZL, Cao W, Biancani P, et al. Nongenomic effects of progesterone on the contraction of muscle cells from the guinea pig colon. Am J Physiol Gastrointest Liver Physiol 2006;290:G1008–15.
60. Pimentel M, Chatterjee S, Chow EJ, et al. Neomycin improves constipation-predominant irritable bowel syndrome in a fashion that is dependent on the presence of methane gas: subanalysis of a double-blind randomized controlled study. Dig Dis Sci 2006;51:1297–301.
61. Pimentel M, Mayer AG, Park S, et al. Methane production during lactulose breath test is associated with gastrointestinal disease presentation. Dig Dis Sci 2003; 48:86–92.
62. Attaluri A, Rao SSC. Is methanogenic flora associated with chronic constipation and altered colonic transit & stool characteristics? Gastroenterology Vol. 132:4(Supp 2:T1945).

63. Pimentel M, Lin HC, Enayati P, et al. Methane, a gas produced by enteric bacteria, slows intestinal transit and augments small intestinal contractile activity. Am J Physiol Gastrointest Liver Physiol 2006;290:G1089–95.

64. Bleijenberg G, Kuijpers HC. Treatment of Spastic Pelvic Floor Syndrome with Biofeedback. Dis Colon Rectum 1987;30:101–11.

65. Duthie GS, Bartolo DCC. Anismus: The Cause of Constipation? Results of Investigation and Treatment. World J Surg 1992;16:831–5.

66. Rao SS, Kavlock R, Rao S. Influence of body position and stool characteristics on defecation in humans. Am J Gastroenterol 2006;101:2790–6.

67. Pinho M, Yoshioka K, Keighley MRB. Long Term Results of Anorectal Myectomy for Chronic Constipation. Br J Surg 1989;76:1163–4.

68. Hallan RI, Williams NS, Melling J, et al. Treatment of Animus in Intractable Constipation with Botulinum A Toxin. Lancet 1988;ii:714–7.

69. Joo JS, Agachan F, Wolff B, et al. Initial North American Experience with Botulinum Toxin Type A for Treatment of Anismus. Dis Colon Rectum 1996;39:1107–11.

70. Heaton KW, Radvan J, Cripps H, et al. Defecation frequency and timing, and stool form in the general population: a prospective study. Gut 1992;33:818–24.

71. O'Donnell LJ, Virjee J, Heaton KW. Detection of pseudodiarrhoea by simple clinical assessment of intestinal transit rate. Bmj 1990;300:439–40.

72. Koch A, Voderholzer WA, Klauser AG, et al. Symptoms in Chronic Constipation. Dis Colon Rectum 1997;40:902–6.

73. Glia A, Lindberg F, L.H, Mihocsa L, et al. Clinical Value of Symptom Assessment in Patients with Constipation. Dis Colon Rectum 1999;42:1401–8.

74. Karasick S, Ehrlich SM. Is constipation a disorder of defecation or impaired motility? distinction based on defecography and colonic transit studies. AJR Am J Roentgenol 1996;166:63–6.

75. Ashraf W, Park F, Quigley EMM, et al. An Examination of the Reliability of Reported Stool Frequency in the Diagnosis of Idiopathic Constipation. Am J Gastroenterol 1996;91:26–32.

76. Metcalf AM, Phillips SF, Zinsmeister AR. Simplified Assessment of Segmental Colonic Transit. Gastroenterology 1987;92:40–7.

77. Ehrenpreis ED, Jorge JMN, Schiano TD, et al. Why Colonic Marker Studies Don't Measure Transit Time. Gastroenterology 1997;110A:728.

78. Rao S. A comparative study of SmartPill® and radioopaque markers for the assessment of colonic transit time in humans. Gastroenterology Vol. 132:4(Supp 2).

79. Rao SSC, Mudipalli RS, Stessman M, et al. Characterization of Manometric Changes in Dyssynergic Defecation (Anismus). Am J Gastroenterol 2001;96:A99.

80. Pelsang RE, Rao SSC, Welcher K. FECOM: A New Artificial Stool for Evaluating Defecation. Am J Gastroenterol 1999;94:183–6.

81. Chaudhary NA, Truelone SC. Human Colonic Motility: A Comparative Study of Normal Subjects, Patients with Ulcerative Colitis and Patients with Irritable Bowel Syndrome. A Resting Pattern of Motility. Gastroenterology 1961;40:11–7.

82. Gertken JT, Cocjin J, Pehlivanov N, et al. Comorbidities associated with constipation in children referred for colon manometry may mask functional diagnoses. J Pediatr Gastroenterol Nutr 2005;41:328–31.

83. Remes-Troche JM, Rao SS. Diagnostic testing in patients with chronic constipation. Curr Gastroenterol Rep 2006;8:416–24.

84. Sackett DL. Rules of evidence and clinical recommendations on the use of antithrombotic agents. Chest 1986;89:2S–3S.

85. Brandt LJ, Schoenfeld P, Prather CM, et al. Evidence-based position statement on the management of chronic constipation in North America. Am J Gastroenterol 2005;100:S1–S22.

86. Ramkumar D, Rao SS. Efficacy and safety of traditional medical therapies for chronic constipation: systematic review. Am J Gastroenterol 2005;100:936–71.

87. Chung BD, Parekh U, Sellin JH. Effect of increased fluid intake on stool output in normal healthy volunteers. J Clin Gastroenterol 1999;28:29–32.

88. Whitehead WE, Drinkwater D, Cheskin LJ, et al. Constipation in the Elderly Living at Home: Definition, Prevalence, and Relationship to Life Style and Health Status. J Am Geriatr Soc 1989;37:423–9.

89. Heaton KW, Wood N, Cripps HA, et al. The Call to Stool and its Relationship to Constipation: A Community Study. Eur J Gast Hepaol 1994;6:145–9.

90. Burkitt DP, Walker ARP, Painter NS. Effect of Dietary Fiber on Stool and Transit Times and its Role in the Causation of Disease. Lancet 1972;ii:1408–11.

91. Tucker DM, Sandstead HH, Logan GM. Dietary Fiber and Personality Factors as Determinants of Stool Output. Gastroenterology 1981;81:879–83.

92. Voderholzer WA, Schatke W, Muhldorfer BE, et al. Clinical Response to Dietary Fiber Treatment of Chronic Constipation. Am J Gastroenterol 1997;92:95–8.

93. Tramonte SM, Brand MB, Mulrow CD, et al. The Treatment of Chronic Constipation in Adults: A Systematic Review. J Gen Intern Med 1997;12:15–24.

94. Kline & Company, Non Prescription Drugs USA 2000; Table 3-3: 44.

95. Lederle FA, Busch DL, Mattox KM, et al. Cost-effective treatment of constipation in the elderly: a randomized double-blind comparison of sorbitol and lactulose. Am J Med 1990;89:597–601.

96. Passmore AP, Davies KW, Flanagan PG, et al. A comparison of Agiolax and lactulose in elderly patients with chronic constipation. Pharmacology 1993; 47(Suppl 1):249–52.

97. DiPalma JA, DeRidder PH, Orlando RC, et al. A randomized, placebo-controlled, multicenter study of the safety and efficacy of a new polyethylene glycol laxative. Am J Gastroenterol 2000;95:446–50.

98. Corazziari E, Badiali D, Habib FI, et al. Small volume isosmotic polyethylene glycol electrolyte balanced solution (PMF-100) in treatment of chronic nonorganic constipation. Dig Dis Sci 1996;41:1636–42.

99. Corazziari E, Badiali D, Bazzocchi G, et al. Long term efficacy, safety, and tolerability of low daily doses of isosmotic polyethylene glycol electrolyte balanced solution (PMF-100) in the treatment of functional chronic constipation. Gut 2000; 46:522–6.

100. Verne GN, Eaker EY, Davis RH, et al. Colchicine is an effective treatment for patients with chronic constipation: an open-label trial. Dig Dis Sci 1997;42:1959–63.

101. Cuppoletti J, Malinowska DH, Tewari KP, et al. SPI-0211 activates T84 cell chloride transport and recombinant human ClC-2 chloride currents. Am J Physiol Cell Physiol 2004;287:C1173–83.

102. Camilleri M, Bharucha AE, Ueno R, et al. Effect of a selective chloride channel activator, lubiprostone, on gastrointestinal transit, gastric sensory, and motor functions in healthy volunteers. Am J Physiol Gastrointest Liver Physiol 2006; 290:G942–7.

103. Johanson JF, Wald A, Tougas G, et al. Effect of tegaserod in chronic constipation: a randomized, double-blind, controlled trial. Clin Gastroenterol Hepatol 2004;2:796–805.

104. Prather CM, Camilleri M, Zinsmeister AR, et al. Tegaserod accelerates orocecal transit in patients with constipation-predominant irritable bowel syndrome. Gastroenterology 2000;118:463–8.
105. Kamm MA, Muller-Lissner S, Talley NJ, et al. Tegaserod for the treatment of chronic constipation: a randomized, double-blind, placebo-controlled multinational study. Am J Gastroenterol 2005;100:362–72.
106. Camilleri M, McKinzie S, Fox J, et al. Effect of renzapride on transit in constipation-predominant irritable bowel syndrome. Clin Gastroenterol Hepatol 2004;2: 895–904.
107. Gonenne J, Camilleri M, Ferber I, et al. Effect of alvimopan and codeine on gastrointestinal transit: a randomized controlled study. Clin Gastroenterol Hepatol 2005;3:784–91.
108. Paulson DM, Kennedy DT, Donovick RA, et al. Alvimopan: an oral, peripherally acting, mu-opioid receptor antagonist for the treatment of opioid-induced bowel dysfunction–a 21-day treatment-randomized clinical trial. J Pain 2005;6:184–92.
109. Camilleri M. Alvimopan, a selective peripherally acting mu-opioid antagonist. Neurogastroenterol Motil 2005;17:157–65.
110. Currie M. Effects of a single dose administration of MD-1100 on safety,tolerability,exposure, and stool consistency in heathy subjects. Am J Gastroenterol 2005;100:S328.
111. Kurtz C. Effects of multi-dose administration of MD-1100 on safety,tolerability,exposure, and pharmacodynamics in healthy subjects. Gastroenterology 2006; 130:A26.
112. Chiarioni G, Whitehead WE, Pezza V, et al. Biofeedback is superior to laxatives for normal transit constipation due to pelvic floor dyssynergia. Gastroenterology 2006;130:657–64.
113. Chiarioni G, Salandini L, Whitehead WE. Biofeedback benefits only patients with outlet dysfunction, not patients with isolated slow transit constipation. Gastroenterology 2005;129:86–97.
114. Rao SS, Seaton K, Miller M, et al. Randomized controlled trial of biofeedback, sham feedback, and standard therapy for dyssynergic defecation. Clin Gastroenterol Hepatol 2007;5:331–8.
115. Lorenzo DIC, Flores AF, Reddy SN, et al. Use of Colonic Manometry to Differentiate Causes of Contractable Constipation in Children. J Pediatr 1992;120: 690–5.
116. Pemberton JH, Rath DM, Ilstrup DM. Evaluation and surgical treatment of severe chronic constipation. Ann Surg 1991;214:403–11, discussion 411–3.
117. Ho YH, Tan M, Eu KW, et al. Laparoscopic-assisted compared with open total colectomy in treating slow transit constipation. Aust N Z J Surg 1997;67:562–5.
118. Nyam DC, Pemberton JH, Ilstrup DM, et al. Long-term results of surgery for chronic constipation. Dis Colon Rectum 1997;40:273–9.

Alterations in the Intestinal Microbiota and Functional Bowel Symptoms

Yehuda Ringel, MD*, Ian M. Carroll, PhD

KEYWORDS

- Functional gastrointestinal disorders • Irritable bowel syndrome
- Intestinal microbiota • Intestinal physiology • Antibiotics
- Probiotics • Lactobacillus • Bifidobacteria

Functional gastrointestinal disorders (FGIDs) are highly prevalent in Western countries with irritable bowel syndrome (IBS) being the most prevalent (10%–20%)[1] and best studied condition. Traditionally, IBS has been considered a disorder arising from an altered brain-gut axis that can be associated with gastrointestinal (GI) hypersensitivity (which may lead to discomfort and pain) and GI motor dysfunction (which may lead to diarrhea, constipation, or alternating bowel movements). Recent studies have implicated new theories that suggest additional ethological factors in the pathogenesis of this disorder. These factors include genetic predeterminants, pathogenic bacterial infection and inflammation, alterations in the normal gut microbiota, food allergy, and an altered gut immune function.[2,3] As IBS is a heterogeneous disorder, it is possible that there are heterogeneous etiologies that may relate to the different clinical subtypes or different subgroups of the disorder. However, despite intensive research over the past few years, the pathophysiology of this disorder is still not clear, and no single ethological factor with a defined pathogenic mechanism has been identified for any form of IBS.

Recent consumer marketing has increased physicians' and patients' interest in using antibiotics and nutritional supplements, such as probiotics, to enhance GI health and relieve the GI symptoms associated with IBS. However, despite supportive clinical data on the use of these products in certain GI diseases, such as infectious, traveler's and antibiotic-associated diarrhea, and some inflammatory bowel disease (IBD) conditions, the clinical data on their use in FGIDs are limited, and the beneficial effect(s) of altering the intestinal flora to alleviate functional bowel symptoms remains undefined/uncertain.

Division of Gastroenterology and Hepatology, University of North Carolina at Chapel Hill School of Medicine, 4107 BioInformatics Building, CB# 7080, 130 Mason Farm Road, Chapel Hill, NC 27599-7080, USA
* Corresponding author.
E-mail address: ringel@med.unc.edu (Y. Ringel).

Gastrointest Endoscopy Clin N Am 19 (2009) 141–150
doi:10.1016/j.giec.2008.12.004
1052-5157/08/$ – see front matter © 2009 Elsevier Inc. All rights reserved.

giendo.theclinics.com

This article discusses the role of GI bacterial flora (microbiota) in the pathophysiology of functional bowel symptoms. We review the existing data on the alterations of the intestinal microbiota in patients with IBS, the effect(s) of these alterations on intestinal physiology, and the clinical data regarding the beneficial effect(s) of manipulation of intestinal microbiota on functional GI symptoms.

ALTERATIONS IN INTESTINAL MICROBIOTA CONTRIBUTE TO FUNCTIONAL BOWEL SYMPTOMS

Indirect evidence that bacteria play a role in IBS comes from epidemiologic, physiologic, and clinical data. Epidemiologic studies have shown that GI infection (eg, acute gastroenteritis) is a strong predictor for the development of IBS.[4] Indeed, up to one-third of patients that recover from an intestinal infection continue to have chronic GI symptoms and may meet the criteria for IBS.[4,5] This suggests that in some patients, IBS can start with an acute infection, leading to an ongoing low level of inflammation or intestinal damage, and then to chronic GI symptoms that persist even after an acute infection has been cleared. This hypothesis is supported by evidence of increased intestinal inflammation associated with IBS, although to a lesser extent than that with IBD.[6–9]

Other epidemiologic studies have documented the presence of small-bowel bacterial overgrowth (SIBO) in a significant portion of IBS patients. The densities of the microbiota in the small intestine are considerably less than those of the colon (1×10^3/ml of luminal contents vs. 1×10^{11}/ml luminal contents, respectively).[10,11] It has been suggested that an increase in the bacterial number in the small intestine can lead to increased fermentation, gas production, and altered gut motility.[12,13] These factors may be responsible, at least in part, for the high prevalence (80%–90%) of abdominal distention, bloating, and gas in patients with IBS.[14] The prevalence of SIBO, diagnosed by hydrogen breath tests in IBS patients, has been found to vary dramatically between studies, ranging from 10% to 84%,[15–17] thus leading to controversy regarding its importance as an ethological factor. Nevertheless, in some studies, eradication of SIBO led to significant improvement in IBS symptoms.

A study in 2008 that developed a novel animal model for IBS has linked two contemporary theories associated with this disorder and implicated the gut microbiota with the genesis of specific IBS symptoms.[18] This study demonstrated that rats infected with Campylobacter jejuni (modeling postinfectious-IBS, [PI-IBS]) resulted in SIBO in 27% of the animals tested. Additionally, altered stool consistency and rectal lymphocytosis were prevalent in these animals with SIBO. This study demonstrates that GI–infection-induced SIBO may lead to persistent inflammation and change in GI function that may have an impact on IBS symptoms.

ALTERATIONS IN INTESTINAL MICROBIOTA AFFECT GI PHYSIOLOGY

Further evidence that the GI microbiota play an important role in IBS comes form studies investigating the effect(s) of intestinal microbiota on the physiology of the GI tract. An altered gut function, both in motility and sensation, is thought to be responsible for most of the bothersome symptoms experienced by patients with IBS. The data available related to the effect(s) of the intestinal microbiota on GI function are drawn mostly from animal studies and a few recent human clinical studies. For example, it has been demonstrated that germ-free rats (rats lacking a normal microbiota) have a profound altered gut motility, including significantly delayed small-bowel transit time and a prolonged interdigestive migratory motor complex (MMC) period.[19] Interestingly, the addition of normal microbiota to these germ-free rats has been shown to increase the small-bowel transit time and the interdigestive MMC. A study in 2001 investigated the effect of specific members of the gut microbiota on gut motility by colonizing germ-free rats with a single/one particular bacterial member of the normal gut microbiota.[20] In this study, germ-free rats that were mono-associated with either *Lactobacillus acidophilus* or *Bifidobacterium bifidum* showed a reduction in their interdigestive MMC period and an increased small-bowel transit time. Moreover, in these mono-association studies it was found that *Escherichia coli* and *Micrococcus luteus* delayed gut motility, demonstrating that different members of the normal gut microbiota have differing effects on intestinal motility.

Additional studies that implicate gut micro-organisms in the genesis of IBS symptoms come form a mouse model that mimics postinfectious IBS. Mice infected with the nematode *Trichinella spiralis* (Tsp) were found to have altered muscle contractility including increased retroperistalsis, reduced overall peristaltic frequency, and altered intestinal sensitivity. These changes persisted for up to 42 days in the absence of overt inflammation.[21,22] These findings are particularly interesting since intestinal dysmotility and altered visceral sensation are implicated in the pathophysiology of IBS. Together, these studies emphasize the importance of a normal intestinal bacterial microbiota in preserving and maintaining normal GI function.

THE INTESTINAL MICROFLORA IN PATIENTS WITH FUNCTIONAL BOWEL DISORDERS DIFFER FROM THOSE IN HEALTHY PERSONS

The intestinal microbiota is a complex community of bacteria, archaea, and eukarya. The bacterial fraction is believed to contain greater than 500 different species and can reach viable numbers of 10^{11} cells per gram of luminal contents,[10] with the highest densities residing in the colon. Greater than 55 bacterial divisions exist, yet only two bacterial divisions (Bacteroidetes and Firmicutes) predominate in the human GI microbiota.[23–25]

Investigating the intestinal microbiota of patients with a specific GI disorder, for example, IBS, poses several significant limitations. First, the complete composition of the GI microbiota remains to be characterized, and the number of bacterial species present in the gut is not yet defined.[26] Thus, at this point, it is impossible to determine the complete differences in the microbiological makeup of a specific population of interest and to fully compare the intestinal microbiota between different populations. The second limitation relates to the heterogeneity of FGIDs. It is not yet clear how many of the different subtypes of these conditions represent actual differences in the underlying pathophysiology. Third, the stability of intestinal microbiota in IBS patients may fluctuate, particularly across different patient populations. For example, a study using molecular techniques demonstrated a considerable instability of the microbiota over time in patients with IBS.[27] Conversely, the structure of the intestinal microbiota of healthy adults has been shown to be consistent over time.[28] Fourth, there is a topographic variability in the GI microbiota in which the bacterial densities and composition differ significantly between the small bowel and large bowel[10,11] and across different sections/parts (ie, proximal versus distal) of the large bowel.[29] Fifth, the bacteria adherent to the intestinal mucosa can differ from those found in the lumen of the gut.[30] Sixth, particularly with respect to IBS, other factors that are hard to control, such as gut motility, diet, and medications, may affect the gut microbiota. Finally, all current methodologies to assess the densities and composition of GI microbiota have inherent limitations. For example, polymerase chain reaction (PCR) based techniques cannot distinguish between live and dead bacteria. Nevertheless, new advances in molecular biology techniques have allowed researchers to carry out more detailed profiling of the gut microbiota that were previously unavailable. Despite these limitations/caveats, several studies have highlighted the differences in the bacterial quality of the adult human intestine between IBS patients and healthy controls.

Early studies using classic culture techniques were limited to a small number of bacteria. Nevertheless, these initial studies found lower levels of coliform bacteria, Lactobacilli, and Bifidobacteria species[31–33] and higher numbers of Clostridium species[34] and Enterobacteriaceae in the feces of patients with IBS compared to those in controls.[32]

New advances in molecular biology, such as quantitative PCR (qPCR),[35] denaturing gradient gel electrophoresis (DGGE) fingerprinting,[27,33] fluorescent in situ hybridization (FISH),[36] and terminal–restriction fragment length polymorphism (T-RFLP) fingerprinting,[37] have aided in the detailed characterization of the microbiota from patients with IBS.

A 2005 study using qPCR[35] assayed the levels of 20 specific bacterial species in stool samples from IBS patients and healthy controls and demonstrated a decrease in the numbers of Lactobacillus species in IBS-D patients and an increase in the number of Veillonella species in IBS-C patients compared with those in healthy controls. In 2006, another study used the sensitive genetic fingerprinting technique DGGE to determine the differences of the overall structure of the gut microbiota in IBS patients and healthy controls.[27] This study demonstrated that the fingerprint profiles of the GI microbiota from IBS patients and healthy controls were unique to each individual. However, the fingerprint profiles generated by DGGE from samples taken 6 months apart from IBS patients displayed more variability when compared with that of samples obtained from healthy controls. These results suggest that the gut microbiota may be less stable over time in patients with IBS.

Despite these studies that associate the gut microbiota with IBS, it is unclear whether the mucosal-adherent and luminal intestinal microbiota differ significantly in these patients. In addition, the relative contribution of these two bacterial populations to the altered physiology and symptom development in IBS remains to be determined. Thus, a 2005 study that analyzed the bacteria adherent to the gut mucosa demonstrated that the density of the bacterial biofilm (a layer of micro-organisms that form a coat on the surface of the intestine) was significantly larger in IBS patients when compared with that in healthy controls, although the biofilm from IBS biopsies were not as dense as those from IBD patients.[36] Moreover, the predominant bacteria adherent to the intestinal mucosa in IBS patients (the *Eubacterium rectale-Clostridium coccoides* group) accounted for 48% of the total adherent bacteria compared with 32% in healthy controls, demonstrating compositional difference in the adherent microbiota between IBS patients and healthy controls.

Another study used a novel approach to analyze the gut microbiota and detect subtle differences in the quality of the gut microbiota between IBS patients and healthy controls.[38] In this approach microbiota DNA obtained from patients experiencing IBS and healthy controls were pooled separately and then fractionated based on the mass of the nucleic acids. Selected fractions where then analyzed by sequencing more than 3,000 16S rDNA genes. Ultimately, it was discovered that the microbiota from IBS patients and healthy controls differed in several bacterial species including Coprococcus spp Collinsella spp and Coprobacillus spp.

Our research group has recently used three methods (conventional culture, qPCR and T-RFLP) to characterize the intestinal microbiota, focusing on patients with IBS-D and comparing it to the intestinal flora of healthy controls. Using conventional culture, we found that there was a significant increase in the number of aerobes in fecal samples from IBS-D patients. Moreover, we have demonstrated a significant differences in the concentrations of Lactobacillus and Bifidobacterium species in the same samples from IBS-D patients compared to healthy controls using qPCR. Furthermore, we have demonstrated a distinct difference in the structure of the gut microbiota between IBS-D patients and healthy controls using T-RFLP.[37]

Collectively, these studies demonstrate distinct differences in the quality, quantity, and temporal stability of the gut microbiota in IBS patients when compared with that in healthy controls. However, the data on this issue are still limited and not consistent. Further studies using novel molecular methods are needed to identify which bacterial divisions/species are deranged in the gut of IBS patients.

CLINICAL DATA ON THE EFFECTS OF MANIPULATION OF THE INTESTINAL MICROBIOTA BY PROBIOTICS AND ANTIBIOTICS

Early studies relating to the clinical use of probiotics as a treatment for IBS have shown mixed results and exhibited considerable methodological limitations.[39] However, in the last 5 years, a number of studies that have employed sound methodologies have provided more solid data regarding the use of certain probiotics for the treatment of IBS. In a study on diarrhea-predominant IBS, 25 patients were randomized to receive either VSL#3 (a probiotic product containing eight species of bacteria, total of 450×10^9 lyophilized bacteria in a sachet) or a placebo twice daily for 8 weeks.[40] The two groups did not differ significantly with regard to global relief of symptoms, bowel function, or mean GI transit measurements; however, the probiotic group had a significant post-treatment reduction in abdominal bloating ($P = 0.046$); whereas, the placebo group did not ($P = 0.54$). This study was followed by a second study targeting IBS patients with predominant symptoms of bloating.[41] Forty-eight patients were randomized to receive either VSL#3 or a placebo for 8 weeks. In this trial, the probiotic mixture significantly reduced flatulence during the treatment period compared with the placebo group ($P<0.01$) but did not significantly alleviate bloating. The mixture of probiotics also slowed colonic transit compared with that in placebo group ($P = 0.05$). Since the product used in these two trials contained eight different bacteria, it is not known which of its probiotic bacterial species (or combination of species) is responsible for the limited effects observed in these small studies.

In 2005, researchers from Europe conducted two relatively large probiotic studies in IBS patients; both studies demonstrated positive effects. In the first study, 77 patients with IBS were randomized to receive malted milk with either *Lactobacillus salivarius* UCC4331 (1×10^{10} live bacterial cells) or *Bifidobacterium infantis* 35624 (1×10^{10} live bacterial cells) or a placebo.[42] After 8 weeks, patients in the *B infantis* group had a greater reduction in most of the study endpoint scores, including symptom composite scores and individual scores, for abdominal pain/discomfort, bloating/distention, and bowel-movement difficulty, when compared with those in patients receiving a placebo. In addition, *B infantis* treatment was associated with normalization of the IL-10/IL-12 ratio in peripheral blood, possibly suggesting an immune-modulating effect. Interestingly, no significant benefits were observed with *L salivarius* over the placebo.

A more recent study further assessed *B infantis* in a multicenter placebo-controlled trial of 362 women with any subtype of IBS. In this study, 362 patients were randomized to either receive *B infantis* (1×10^6, 1×10^8, or 1×10^{10} colony forming units [CFUs]) or a placebo for 4 weeks.[43] By the end of treatment, the 1×10^8 dose of *B infantis* was more effective ($P<0.05$) than the other doses and the placebo at reducing abdominal pain, symptom composite scores, and individual scores for bloating, bowel dysfunction, incomplete evacuation, straining, and the passage of gas. The overall clinical effect of the 1×10^8 dose of *B infantis* was modest but statistically significant. The other two doses were not significantly better than the placebo. The lack of benefit with the higher dose (1×10^{10} CFU) was most likely related to a technical problem with this formulation, which coagulated into a gluey mass limiting its dissolution and bioavailability.

In 2007/8 we investigated the effect of the probiotic bacteria *Lactobacillus acidophilus* NCFM (L-NCFM) and *Bifidobacterium lactis Bi-07* (B-LBi07) in patients with non-constipation functional bowel disorders. A total of 57 patients were randomized to receive either L-NCFM and B-LBi07 (1×10^{11} CFU total probiotic bacteria) or a placebo twice daily for 8 weeks. We found that supplementation of the diet with these bacteria significantly improved bloating and distention symptoms compared with the placebo ($P = 0.03$).[44] In another study, we demonstrated that daily consumption of a yogurt containing the probiotic bacterium *Bifidobacterium animalis ssp. lactis* Bb12 and the prebiotic inulin was associated with a significant increase in colonic transit compared with placebo ($P = 0.016$).[45]

Several studies have investigated the use of antibiotics in patients with functional bowel disorders and demonstrated some clinical benefit in alleviating functional bowel symptoms, mostly bloating symptoms and gas. Early studies focused on the use of antibiotics in relation to SIBO (diagnosed by hydrogen breath test) in patients with IBS and attributed the observed improvement in functional symptoms primarily to the eradication of SIBO in these patients.[15] Several studies in 2006 showed possible beneficial effects of antibiotics in reducing functional GI symptoms regardless of the presence of abnormal hydrogen breath test.[46,47] A clinical trial in 2008 investigated the effect of rifaximin treatment (550 mg twice daily for 14 days) in 388 patients with D-IBS. This study found a greater relief of global IBS symptoms and bloating in the treatment group (n = 191) over the placebo group (n = 197)[48] primarily in the subgroups of patients with mild-to-moderate abdominal pain or bloating at baseline.[49] Interestingly, the beneficial effect observed at the end of the 2-week treatment period was maintained at the 12-week follow-up period.

Taken together, the results of these studies support the idea that manipulation of the intestinal flora by probiotics or antibiotics may be beneficial in reducing symptoms in some patients with IBS. They also demonstrate that intestinal bacterial modifications can affect aspects of intestinal physiology (eg, intestinal transit time and possibly intestinal immune function) relevant to functional GI disorders.

SUMMARY

Epidemiological data have provided indirect evidence that alterations in the gut microbiota, specifically in association with clinical conditions such as SIBO and PI-IBS, can lead to the generation of functional GI symptoms. Additionally, clinical data have provided evidence that the gut microbiota can affect intestinal physiology (with respect to motility, sensation, and immune function). Furthermore, laboratory research has demonstrated that the GI microbiota in a patient experiencing IBS is distinct from the microbiota harbored within humans and animals with a healthy gut. Taken together these emerging data support the hypothesis that alterations in the intestinal microbiota may have an important role in the pathogenesis of IBS and possibly other functional bowel disorders.

However, considering the complexity of the microbiota and its close inter-relationship with the intestinal intraluminal environment and various host factors, the interpretation of the accumulating data with regard to a possible association between intestinal microbiota and the intestinal function and functional symptoms should be carried out with great caution. For example, it is difficult to establish whether the observed differences in the GI microbiota between IBS patients and healthy controls are a cause of the disorder(s) or an effect of the altered intestinal function or luminal environment in these disorders. The different bacterial species harbored within the microbiota can react differently to changes in multiple/various environmental factors. Small changes in the motility of the gut may have a profound effect on the composition of both the mucosal-adherent and luminal microbiota by simply increasing or reducing the transit time of nonresident bacteria in the intestine and the exposure time that the microbiota would have with consumed nutrients. Alternatively, changes in the redox potential in the gut could lead to a decrease in the densities of aerobic organisms and a subsequent increase in the number of anaerobic organisms in the gut. Thus, the observed changes in the gut microbiota may be a result of a change in the GI function and/or intraluminal environment.

Table 1
Techniques used to assess the differences in the quality and quantity of specific members of the gut microbiota between IBS patients and healthy controls

Reference	IBS Subtype	Method	Clinical Outcome
Balsari et al 1982[31]	Undefined subtype	Culture	↓ coliforms, *Lactobacilli* spp and *Bifidobacteria* spp in IBS patients
Si et al 2004[32]	Undefined subtype	Culture	↓ *Bifidobacteria* spp and an ↑ *Enterobacteriaceae* spp in all IBS patients.
Mättö et al 2005[33]	IBS-D ($n = 12$), IBS-C ($n = 9$), IBS-M ($n = 5$).	Culture & DGGE	↑ total number of aerobes in IBS patients. Temporal instability in IBS patients revealed by DGGE.
Malinen et al 2005[35]	IBS-D ($n = 12$), IBS-C ($n = 9$), IBS-M ($n = 6$).	qPCR	↓ amounts of *Lactobacillus* spp in IBS-D patients. ↑ amounts of *Veillonella* spp in IBS-C patients.
Swidsinski et al 2005[36]	Undefined subtype	FISH	*Eubacterium-Clostridium coccoides* groups accounted for > 40% of the mucosal biofilm compared with <15% in healthy controls.
Kassinen et al 2007[38]	IBS-D ($n = 10$), IBS-C ($n = 8$), IBS-M ($n = 6$).	Nucleic Acid fractionation and sequencing	Significant differences in the levels of *Coprococcus, Collinsella,* and *Coprobacillus* species between IBS patients and healthy controls.

Nevertheless, the epidemiological data on the association between events altering the intestinal microbiota and the development of functional GI symptoms and the exciting reports of derangements in the gut microbial in patients with FGIDs have led to the development of novel approaches for the treatment of these disorders by manipulating the intestinal flora using antibiotics or probiotics. Although the data on the use of antibiotics or probiotics in the treatment of functional bowel disorders are not yet conclusive, the positive results in some of these studies are encouraging and emphasize the need for further research in this area. It is hoped that this may lead to a better understanding of the disorder and the development of new and effective modes of treatments (**Table 1**).

REFERENCES

1. Longstreth GF, Thompson WG, Chey WD, et al. Functional bowel disorders. In: Drossman DA, Corazziari E, Delvaux M, et al, editors. Rome III: the functional gastrointestinal disorders, 3rd edition. McLean (VA): Degnon Associates; 2006;9:487–555.
2. Azpiroz F, Bouin M, Camilleri M, et al. Mechanisms of hypersensitivity in IBS and functional disorders. Neurogastroenterol Motil 2007;19(Suppl 1):62–88.
3. Ringel Y, Drossman DA. Irritable bowel syndrome. In: Runge MS, Greganti MA, editors. Netter's textbook of internal medicine. 2nd edition. Philadelphia: Saunders Elsevier; 2008:59:419–25.
4. Rodriguez AL, Ruigomez A. Increased risk of irritable bowel syndrome after bacterial gastroenteritis: cohort study. BMJ 1999;318:565–6.
5. Spiller RC. Postinfectious irritable bowel syndrome. Gastroenterology 2003;124:1662–71.
6. Quigley EMM. Irritable bowel syndrome and inflammatory bowel disease: interrelated diseases? Chin J Dig Dis 2005;6:122–32.
7. Shulman RJ, Eakin MN, Czyzewski DI, et al. Increased gastrointestinal permeability and gut inflammation in children with functional abdominal pain and irritable bowel syndrome. J Pediatr 2008;153:646–50.
8. Aerssens J, Camilleri M, Talloen W, et al. Alterations in mucosal immunity identified in the colon of patients with irritable bowel syndrome. Clin Gastroenterol Hepatol 2008;6(2):194–205.
9. Ohashi K, Sato Y, Kawai M, et al. Abolishment of TNBS-induced visceral hypersensitivity in mast cell deficient rats. Life Sci 2008;82(7–8):419–23.
10. Whitman WB, Coleman DC, Wiebe WJ. Prokaryotes: the unseen majority. Proc Natl Acad Sci U S A 1998;95:6578–83.
11. Othman M, Agüero R, Lin HC. Alterations in intestinal microbial flora and human disease. Curr Opin Gastroenterol 2008;24(1):11–6.
12. Lin HC. Small intestinal bacterial overgrowth: a framework for understanding irritable bowel syndrome. JAMA 2004;292:852–8.
13. Lee HR, Pimentel M. Bacteria and irritable bowel syndrome: the evidence for small intestinal bacterial overgrowth. Curr Gastroenterol Rep 2006;8:305–11.
14. Ringel Y, Williams RE, Kalilani L, et al. The prevalence, characteristics and impact of bloating symptoms in patients with irritable bowel syndrome. Clinical Gastroenterology and Hepatology, 2009;7:68–72.
15. Pimentel M, Chow EJ, Lin HC. Eradication of small intestinal bacterial overgrowth reduces symptoms of irritable bowel syndrome. Am J Gastroenterol 2000;95:3503–6.

16. Pimentel M, Chow EJ, Lin HC. Normalization of lactulose breath testing correlates with symptom improvement in irritable bowel syndrome. A double-blind, randomized, placebo-controlled study. Am J Gastroenterol 2003;98:412–9.
17. McCallum R, Schultz C, Sostarich S. Evaluating the role of small intestinal bacterial overgrowth (SIBO) in diarrhea predominant IBS (IBS-D) patients utilizing the glucose breath test. Gastroenterology 2005;128:T1118.
18. Pimentel M, Chatterjee S, Chang C, et al. A new rat model links two contemporary theories in irritable bowel syndrome. Dig Dis Sci 2008;53(4):982–9.
19. Caenepeel P, Janssens J, Vantrappen G, et al. Interdigestive myoelectric complex in germ-free rats. Dig Dis Sci 1989;34(8):1180–4.
20. Husebye E, Hellström PM, Sundler F, et al. Influence of microbial species on small intestinal myoelectric activity and transit in germ-free rats. Am J Physiol Gastrointest Liver Physiol 2001;280(3):G368–80.
21. Barbara G, Vallance BA, Collins SM. Persistent intestinal neuromuscular dysfunction after acute nematode infection in mice. Gastroenterology 1997;113(4):1224–32.
22. Bercik P, Wang L, Verdu EF, et al. Visceral hyperalgesia and intestinal dysmotility in a mouse model of postinfective gut dysfunction. Gastroenterology 2004;127:179–87.
23. Bäckhed F, Ley RE, Sonnenburg JL, et al. Host-bacterial mutualism in the human intestine. Science 2005;307(5717):1915–20.
24. Ley RE, Turnbaugh PJ, Klein S, et al. Human gut microbes associated with obesity. Nature 2006;444(7122):1022–3.
25. Gill SR, Pop M, Deboy RT, et al. Metagenomic analysis of the human distal gut microbiome. Science 2006;312(5778):1355–9.
26. Peterson DA, Frank DN, Pace NR, et al. Metagenomic approaches for defining the pathogenesis of inflammatory bowel diseases. Cell Host Microbe 2008;3:417–27.
27. Maukonen J, Mättö J, Satokari R, et al. PCR DGGE and RT-PCR DGGE show diversity and short-term temporal stability in the Clostridium coccoides-Eubacterium rectale group in the human intestinal microbiota. Microb Ecol 2006;58(3):517–28.
28. Tannock GW, Munro K, Harmsen HJ, et al. Analysis of the fecal microflora of human subjects consuming a probiotic product containing *Lactobacillus rhamnosus* DR20. Appl Environ Microbiol 2000;66:2578–88.
29. Bibiloni R, Mangold M, Madsen KL, et al. The bacteriology of biopsies differs between newly diagnosed, untreated, Crohn's disease and ulcerative colitis patients. J Med Microbiol 2006;55(8):1141–9.
30. Zoetendal EG, von Wright A, Vilpponen-Salmela T, et al. Mucosa-associated bacteria in the human gastrointestinal tract are uniformly distributed along the colon and differ from the community recovered from feces. Appl Environ Microbiol 2002;68(7):3401–7.
31. Balsari A, Ceccarelli A, Dubini F, et al. The fecal microbial population in irritable bowel syndrome. Microbiologica 1982;5:185–94.
32. Si JM, Yu YC, Fan YJ, et al. Intestinal microecology and quality of life in irritable bowel syndrome patients. World J Gastroenterol 2004;10:1802–5.
33. Mättö J, Maunuksela L, Kajander K, et al. Composition and temporal stability of gastrointestinal microbiota in irritable bowel syndrome–a longitudinal study in IBS and control subjects. FEMS Immunol Med Microbiol 2005;43(2):213–22.
34. Bradley HK, Wyatt GM, Bayliss CE, et al. Instability in the faecal flora of a patient suffering from food-related irritable bowel syndrome. J Med Microbiol 1987;23:29–32.

35. Malinen E, Rinttilä T, Kajander K, et al. Analysis of the fecal microbiota of irritable bowel syndrome patients and healthy controls with real-time PCR. Am J Gastroenterol 2005;100(2):373–82.
36. Swidsinski A, Weber J, Loening-Baucke V, et al. Spatial organization and composition of the mucosal flora in patients with inflammatory bowel disease. J Clin Microbiol 2005;43(7):3380–9.
37. Carroll I, Xiang JS, Keku TO, et al. Microbiological characterization of stool samples from patients with diarrhea predominant irritable bowel syndrome (D-IBS). Gastroenterology 2008;134(4 Suppl 1):A681.
38. Kassinen A, Krogius-Kurikka L, Mäkivuokko H, et al. The fecal microbiota of irritable bowel syndrome patients differs significantly from that of healthy subjects. Gastroenterology 2007;133(1):24–33.
39. Quigley EM. Probiotics in functional gastrointestinal disorders: what are the facts? Curr Opin Pharmacol 2008;8:704–8.
40. Kim HJ, Camilleri M, McKinzie S, et al. A randomized controlled trial of a probiotic, VSL#3, on gut transit and symptoms in diarrhoea-predominant irritable bowel syndrome. Aliment Pharmacol Ther 2003;17:895–904.
41. Kim HJ, Vazquez Roque MI, Camilleri M, et al. A randomized controlled trial of a probiotic combination VSL#3 and placebo in irritable bowel syndrome with bloating. Neurogastroenterol Motil 2005;17:687–96.
42. O'Mahoney L, McCarthy J, Kelly P, et al. Lactobacillus and bifidobacterium in irritable bowel syndrome: symptom responses and relationship to cytokine profiles. Gastroenterology 2005;128:541–51.
43. Whorwell PJ, Altringer L, Morel J, et al. Efficacy of an encapsulated probiotic Bifidobacterium infantis 35624 in women with irritable bowel syndrome. Am J Gastroenterol 2006;101:1581–90.
44. Ringel Y, Palsson OS, Leyer G, et al. Probiotic bacteria Lactobacillus Acidophilus Ncfm and Bifidobacterium lactis Bi07 improve symptoms of bloating in patients with functional bowel disorders (FBD). Gastroenterology 2008;134(4 Suppl 1): A549.
45. Ringel-Kulka T, Palsson OS, Maier D, et al. Yogurt containing the probiotic bacteria Bifidobacterium lactis Bb12 and prebiotic inulin significantly improves colonic transit time in subjects with functional bowel symptoms. Am J Gastroenterol 2008;103(S1):S479.
46. Sharara AI, Aoun E, Abdul-Baki H, et al. A randomized double-blind placebo-controlled trial of rifaximin in patients with abdominal bloating and flatulence. Am J Gastroenterol 2006;101(2):326–33.
47. Pimentel M, Chatterjee S, Chow EJ, et al. Neomycin improves constipation-predominant irritable bowel syndrome in a fashion that is dependent on the presence of methane gas: subanalysis of a double-blind randomized controlled study. Dig Dis Sci 2006;51:1297–301.
48. Lembo A, Zakko S, Ferreira N, et al. Rifaximin for the treatment of diarrhea-associated irritable bowel syndrome: short term treatment leading to long term sustained response. Gastroenterology 2008;134(4 Suppl 1):A545.
49. Ringel Y, Zakko S, Ferreira N, et al. Predictors of clinical response from a phase 2 multi-center efficacy trial using rifaximin, a gut-selective, nonabsorbed antibiotic for the treatment of diarrhea-associated irritable bowel syndrome. Gastroenterology 2008;134(4 Suppl 1):A550.

Psychopharmacologic and Behavioral Treatments for Functional Gastrointestinal Disorders

Madhusudan Grover, MD[a], Douglas A. Drossman, MD[b],*

KEYWORDS

- Functional gastrointestinal disorders
- Irritable bowel syndrome • Psychopharmacologic agents
- Behavioral treatments • Brain-gut axis • Treatments

Functional gastrointestinal disorders (FGIDs) are best conceptualized with a biopsychosocial model in which psychosocial factors in addition to GI physiologic factors contribute to the experience of the illness and subsequent behaviors.[1] Modalities such as brain imaging and neurotransmitter research demonstrate that FGID symptoms result physiologically from a dysregulated brain-gut axis.[2,3] For example, neurotransmitters such as serotonin (5-hydroxytryptamine [5-HT]), norepinephrine (NE), corticotropin releasing factor, and opioids, among others, modify both motility and sensation in the gut. This has made psychopharmacologic and behavioral therapies particularly attractive treatment strategies. Their benefit also lies in managing associated psychological disturbances commonly associated with FGIDs.[4] The use of psychotropic agents for FGIDs has grown significantly in the last 2 decades. At least 1 in 8 patients with irritable bowel syndrome (IBS) is offered an antidepressant.[5] In addition, behavioral treatments are an area of increasing research and practice in the management of FGIDs, especially at the severe and refractory end of the spectrum. However, proper treatment is challenging due to insufficient understanding of

---

All authors report no conflict of interest with regard to financial interests or affiliations with institutions, organizations, or companies as related to this manuscript, and no products or services are discussed.

[a] Division of Internal Medicine, Michigan State University, B-301 Clinical Center, East Lansing, MI 48824, USA

[b] UNC Center for Functional GI and Motility Disorders, 4150 Bioinformatics Building CB#7080, University of North Carolina, Chapel Hill, NC 27599-7080, USA

* Corresponding author.

E-mail address: drossman@med.unc.edu (D.A. Drossman).

Gastrointest Endoscopy Clin N Am 19 (2009) 151–170
doi:10.1016/j.giec.2008.12.001
1052-5157/08/$ – see front matter © 2009 Elsevier Inc. All rights reserved.

giendo.theclinics.com

the complex nature of these disorders, lack of well-designed drug studies, and variability among the treatment efficacy end-points. In addition, lack of therapists in the community dealing with GI disorders makes behavioral treatments less approachable. Lastly, there is insufficient understanding and knowledge of these disorders among physicians and specialists in primary care, which hinders early and effective approach to management.

We discuss the rationale, mechanisms, efficacy, and practical aspects of psychopharmacologic, behavioral, and combination treatments in the management of FGIDs with a focus on some of the more recent work in this field.

RATIONALE FOR THE USE OF PSYCHOPHARMACOLOGIC AND BEHAVIORAL TREATMENTS

The most commonly used psychotropic agents for FGIDs are antidepressants, especially tricyclic antidepressants (TCAs). The rationale for their use in FGIDs is highlighted in **Box 1**. Several reviews and meta-analyses have shown that antidepressants achieve both pain reduction and global symptom improvement in IBS and other FGIDs.[6] Notably, the analgesic effect appears independent of the actions on mood disturbance, and it occurs before improvement in psychological symptoms.[7,8]

Second, in higher dosages, these agents treat psychiatric diagnoses such as depression or anxiety disorder or psychological distress, which, in turn, can improve global symptoms and health-related quality of life (HRQOL). However, clinical improvement with antidepressants, though correlated with psychological scores, is independent of psychological improvement.[7] This indicates a separate but complementary mechanism of action, that is, central analgesia, over treatment of mood disturbance with these agents.

Finally, and in addition to their central effects on mood and pain modulation, these agents also affect gut motility. TCAs with NE and anticholinergic action show a prolongation of the orocecal transit time, thus improving diarrhea symptoms.[7,9] In contrast, selective serotonin reuptake inhibitors (SSRIs) reduce orocecal transit time, which may help constipation-predominant symptoms.[9]

The rationales for the use of behavioral treatments relate primarily to modifying maladaptive cognitions (ie, persistent thoughts and beliefs) or behaviors that impair

---

Box 1
Potential benefits for use of psychopharmacologic agents in FGIDs

Central effects:

1. Alters central pain perception—analgesia or antihyperalgesia

2. Therapeutic effects on mood—to manage general anxiety, hypervigilance, symptom-related anxiety, agoraphobia, and increased stress responsiveness

3. Treatment of associated psychiatric disorders—depression, posttraumatic stress disorder (PTSD), somatization

4. Treatment of associated sleep disturbances

Peripheral effects:

1. Peripheral analgesic effects—alters visceral afferent signaling

2. Effect in GI physiology (motility and secretion) via effects on cholinergic, noradrenergic, and serotonergic pathways

3. Smooth muscle effects on viscera—for example, gastric fundic relaxation

clinical recovery. These treatments are different from "talk therapy," that is, exploratory or analytically oriented psychological treatments, as they focus on the "here and now" to help patients adapt to the condition. The potential targets for behavioral treatments are listed in **Box 2**. These treatments can be successful with or without improvement in pain and other symptoms; they can lead to improved clinical outcomes including HRQOL, daily functioning, and overall satisfaction with treatment. The benefits can occur even in patients without psychiatric comorbidities or mood disturbances,[10] as they seek to target maladaptive beliefs and behaviors and reduce an overactive stress response as well as possibly improve peripheral sensory and motor disturbances commonly seen in patients with severe FGIDs.[11,12] Systematic reviews and meta-analyses have found support for psychological therapies,[6,13] although many of these studies have methodological deficiencies.[14]

ROLE OF PSYCHOLOGICAL FACTORS

Psychosocial factors play a vital role in the natural history of FGIDs, being responsible for predisposition, precipitation, and perpetuation of symptoms and illness behavior. Up to three-fourths of FGID patients seeking care at tertiary care referral centers meet diagnostic criteria for a psychiatric disorder, the most common being anxiety and depression,[15] though in general the prevalence is much lower for patients seen in primary care or even general gastroenterology practice.[16] A history of major life events such as sexual abuse, other life stress, maladaptive coping (catastrophizing), or psychological distress is common in IBS, particularly for patients with more severe symptoms, and such problems perpetuate the severity via maladaptive illness behavior.[17,18] Abuse, life stress, and poor coping can directly affect symptom severity, health care use, HRQOL, and response to treatment.[19] Distress in response to the GI condition can have adverse effects on psychological state or health status independent of there being a specific psychiatric diagnosis. Furthermore, a negative workup, incomplete understanding, and an unsatisfactory explanation from the physician lead to constant worry, fear, and anxiety, and this situation often perpetuates the symptom severity.[20] Postinfectious (PI)-IBS provides an ideal example of psychological factors' influence on IBS disease process.[21] Psychosocial distress at the time of infection has been shown to be an independent predictor of later development of PI-IBS. Stress has been proposed to act by an overarching effect on inflammation and brain-gut axis in PI-IBS.

In addition, there is a subgroup of IBS patients, particularly with more severe illness, that report many non-GI symptoms, and some investigators have hypothesized the existence of broader neurophysiologic processes (eg, so called "somatization") in up to 15% to 45% of IBS patients.[22] In effect, these patients have central

---

Box 2
Targets for behavioral treatments in FGIDs

1. To establish a rational model of illness—reframe maladaptive beliefs

2. To reduce overresponsiveness to stress—for example, stress and autonomic reactivity

3. To reduce or modify maladaptive psychological responses—catastrophizing, symptom-specific anxiety, and shame or guilt

4. To reduce or modify maladaptive behaviors—for example, agoraphobia, seeking diagnostic studies

dysregulation of pain-regulatory pathways[23] and often have comorbid problems such as fibromyalgia, chronic fatigue, or PTSD. This understanding has important implications on using centrally acting treatments alone or in combination to target this broader polysymptomatic process with FGIDs and even predicting response to these agents. These individuals may set lower thresholds for symptom reporting and thus report many symptoms throughout their lives or in response to acute (eg, war, abuse) trauma,[24] and this pattern of symptoms has been shown to respond poorly to peripherally based pharmacologic intervention.[25]

PSYCHOPHARMACOLOGIC AGENTS
General Approach

The IBS and other FGIDs exist across a wide spectrum of severity. On one end are patients with mild to moderate symptoms who can be successfully treated with education, dietary and lifestyle modifications, and gut acting agents (eg, anticholinergics, peripheral 5-HT agents). On the opposite end are the 20% of patients who suffer from severe FGIDs characterized by increased levels of pain, poorer HRQOL, higher levels of health care use, more psychosocial difficulties, and a higher frequency of psychiatric comorbidities. Because these patients are refractory to first- and second-line therapies,[19] they require a multimodal approach in which behavioral tools (eg, cognitive-behavioral treatment, hypnosis, stress management/relaxation) and psychotropic agents are also needed. Notably, many of these treatments can be used in addition to gut acting agents.

An effective physician–patient relationship is the key in the management of FGIDs. A treatment algorithm is depicted in **Fig. 1** for all levels of severity, whereas the centrally acting treatments are mostly used for the moderate to severe end of the spectrum, as noted above. To assure treatment adherence with psychotropic agents, the physician needs to clarify to the patient that these are "central analgesics" and not simply drugs for psychiatric conditions; they have independent effects on pain and can be used in lower dosages than those used to treat major depression. **Box 3** describes an approach to the treatment of FGIDs with psychopharmacologic agents. The choice of the agent depends on specific symptoms targeted, side-effect profile, and past experience with antidepressants. The therapeutic benefit may take 4 to 6 weeks to achieve; however, side effects may be reported within 1 to 2 weeks.[26] Starting at a low dose and a closer follow-up, especially in the first week, may increase compliance. Some of the issues with prescribing these agents are a suboptimal dose or failure to escalate dose if the response is poor, nonadherence, or delayed response.[5] Depending on the response and side effects, another agent with a different mechanism of action can be added to augment treatment efficacy and minimize side effects. Patients with a good response can be successfully maintained on antidepressants for months to years. In addition, patients need to be informed that these agents are not "mind altering," are not addicting, and can be stopped without major withdrawal effects if needed.

Failure to maintain treatment occurs in nearly a quarter of outpatients given antidepressants for FGIDs.[27] Somatization features[22] and the presence of depression[7] or anxiety most significantly interfered with treatment by predicting side effects, poor treatment response, and premature discontinuation. Patients less likely to have a good outcome particularly with TCAs are those with constipation-predominant IBS (IBS-C) or delayed GI motility or patients with medical comorbidities exacerbated by antidepressants and patients with somatization disorder.[7,28] Management algorithms should include specific strategies targeted at patients with these risk

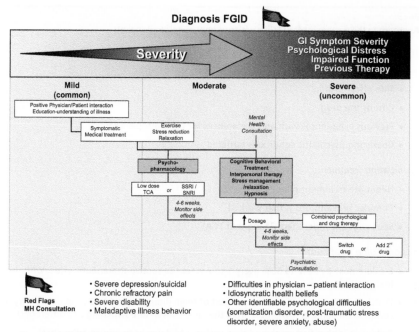

Fig. 1. Treatment algorithm for patients with functional gastrointestinal disorders (FGIDs). Red flags are indications for considering early referral to a mental health professional. There is a range of intensity in psychological approaches to treatment, and intensity of treatment is matched with the severity of FGID.

factors for poor treatment adherence.[29] Class effects of antidepressants are summarized in **Table 1**.

Tricyclic Antidepressants

TCAs are the most rigorously studied class of psychotropic agents used in FGIDs. The results of some of the randomized controlled trials (RCTs) are summarized in **Table 2**. The reason for marginal intention to treat effects in our large study was because one-fourth of the patients dropped out from the treatment arm primarily due to side effects. However, a per-protocol post hoc analysis showed a 20% effect size margin.[7] Clouse and colleagues reported managing 138 IBS patients with antidepressants in whom TCAs were used 130 times, newer agents 39 times, and anxiolytics 47 times. Improvement occurred in 89% and complete remission in 61% of patients.[30] For the most part, despite methodological problems in designing good studies with antidepressants, there is evidence of treatment benefit with TCAs provided patients are able to stay on medication.

TCAs reduce pain sensitivity in chronic neuropathic animal models more effectively than SSRIs.[31] In animal studies, they reduce the frequency of nerve impulses evoked by noxious distension in the colon.[32] The analgesic properties are also likely contributed by alpha-adrenergic, sodium channel blockade, and N-methyl D-aspartate (NMDA) antagonist-like action.[31,33] Their effects on visceral perception have been mixed.[34] A recent study showed that TCAs do not have significant effects on gastric motor function or satiation post nutrient challenge in healthy individuals.[35]

Box 3
Approach to the management of FGIDs with psychopharmacologic agents

1. *Choice of the agent:*
   - Specific symptom treated
   - Side-effect profile
   - Cost of the drug
   - Previous experiences with and preferences for psychotropic agents
   - Coexisting psychiatric conditions targeted

2. *Initiating treatment:*
   - Negotiate treatment plan
   - Consider previous drugs that worked
   - Start with a low dose (eg, 25 mg/d of TCA)

3. *Continuing treatment:*
   - Escalate dose by 25% to 50% every 1 to 2 weeks to receive therapeutic effect with the least possible dose.
   - Watch for side effects. Counsel that most of them disappear in 1 to 2 weeks. If not, try to continue the same or lower dose from the same class before switching to a different class.
   - Follow up within first week and then within 2 to 3 weeks to ensure adherence.
   - Gauge treatment benefit with improvement in coping, daily function, QOL, and emotional state.
   - If there is poor initial response:
     - Readdress patient concerns
     - Switch to a different class
     - Combination therapies (eg, SSRI+TCA, pharmacologic and psychological treatment)
     - If needed, psychiatry consultation for pharmacotherapy
   - Increase doses up to full psychiatric doses if patient can tolerate before discontinuing.
   - If there is no benefit in 6 to 8 weeks on higher doses, alternate strategies (eg, adding psychological treatment or referral) should be sought.
   - Depending on the response and side effects, another agent with different mechanism of action can be added to augment treatment efficacy and minimize side effects.

4. *Stopping treatment:* Continue treatment at minimum effective doses for 6 to 12 months. Long-term therapy may be warranted for some patients. Gradually taper to prevent withdrawal symptoms.

The lack of substantive data on peripheral analgesic properties of TCAs in humans suggests that the more pronounced effects are on central pain modulation. In functional MRI studies, the mid cingulate cortex (MCC) is activated during painful rectal distensions in IBS patients. This activation is associated with poor clinical status in severe IBS, and there is reduced activation with clinical improvement.[36] Those with IBS and abuse report more pain, greater MCC activation, and reduced activity of anterior cingulate cortex (ACC), which is implicated in pain inhibition and arousal.[37]

Table 1 Class effects of psychotropic agents			
	TCAs	SSRIs	SNRIs
Agents	Amitriptyline Imipramine Doxepin Desipramine Nortriptyline	Fluoxetine Sertraline Paroxetine Citalopram Escitalopram	Duloxetine Venlafaxine Desvenlafaxine — —
Dose range	10–200 mg —	10–100 mg —	30–90 mg (duloxetine) 75–225 mg (venlafaxine)
Potential benefits			
• Peripheral pain modulation	++	?	++
• Central antinociception	+++	+	+++ (higher doses of venlafaxine)
• Anxiolysis	+	+++	+
• Motility	++	+	?
• Visceral pain	+++	?	?
• Sleep	++	–	?
• Psychiatric comorbidities	++ (high doses)	+++	+++
Adverse effects	Sedation Constipation Dry mouth/eyes Weight gain Hypotension Sexual dysfunction	Insomnia Diarrhea Night sweats Weight loss Agitation Sexual dysfunction	Nausea Agitation Dizziness Fatigue Liver dysfunction —
Time to action	Few days–2 wk (low doses) 2–6 wk (high doses)	3–6 wk —	3–6 wk —
Efficacy	Good	Moderate	Not adequately studied
Dose adjustments	Common	Usually not needed	Common

Abbreviations: SNRIs, serotonin-norepinephrine reuptake inhibitors; SSRIs, selective serotonin re-uptake inhibitors; TCAs, tricyclic antidepressants.

Furthermore, amitriptyline reduced brain activation during pain in the perigenual (limbic) ACC and parietal association cortex during stress.[38]

Side effects depend on the class of TCAs but for the most part include sedation and anticholinergic (constipation, tachycardia, urinary retention, and xerostomia) and central nervous system (CNS) side effects (insomnia, agitation, and nightmares). TCAs can slow both small-bowel and colonic transit.[9] However, the side-effect profiles vary because of differences in the postsynaptic receptor affinities. In general, secondary amine TCAs (eg, desipramine, nortriptyline) are better tolerated than tertiary amine TCAs (eg, amitriptyline, imipramine) because of their lower antihistaminic and anticholinergic properties.[5]

Table 2
Recent studies on use of TCAs in FGIDs

Citation	Drug	Sample	Study Design	Outcome
Drossman et al, 2003[7]	Desipramine	Women; moderate to severe IBS (n = 431)	12 wk Multicenter, comparator controlled RCT	1. Per-protocol analysis: desipramine superior to placebo; intention-to-treat analysis: not significant. 2. With dosages up to 150 mg, there is no relationship between total dose or plasma level and the clinical response[82]
Otaka et al, 2005[83]	Amitriptyline	Refractory functional dyspepsia(n = 14)	4 wk Double-blind RCT	1. Amitriptyline showed 66.7% efficacy in famotidine-failed group and 75.0% efficacy in the mosapride-failed group.
Morgan et al, 2005[38]	Amitriptyline	Women with severe IBS (n = 19)	4 wk RCT	1. During Stress, amitriptyline reduced pain-related cerebral activations in the perigenual ACC and the left posterior parietal cortex.
Vahedi et al, 2008[84]	Amitriptyline	IBS-D (n = 50)	8 wk Double-blind RCT	1. Lower incidence of loose stool and feeling of incomplete defecation. 2. Increased report of "loss of all symptoms" compared with placebo (68% vs 28%).
Bahar et al, 2008[85]	Amitriptyline	Adolescents IBS (n = 33)	13-wk Double blind RCT	1. Improved overall QOL. 2. Reduction in IBS diarrhea. 3. Improved abdominal pain.

Abbreviations: ACC, anterior cingulate cortex; FGIDs, functional gastrointestinal disorders; IBS, irritable bowel syndrome; RCT, randomized controlled trial; TCAs, tricyclic antidepressants.

Selective Serotonin Reuptake Inhibitors

The main action of SSRIs is to selectively inhibit the reuptake of 5-HT and block the 5-HT transporter protein at the level of presynaptic nerve endings, increasing synaptic concentration of 5-HT. These agents have effects on animal somatic pain models, although the effects are weaker than those of the TCAs.[31] Data on visceral pain perception with SSRIs are mixed, and central nociceptive effects of SSRIs have not been studied. **Table 3** summarizes some of the recent RCTs on use of SSRIs in FGIDs.

SSRIs can be used to augment the overall benefit of TCAs through their effect on anxiety or in sufficient dosages in treating psychiatric comorbidities. Although they are reported to show analgesic effect in neuropathic pain, back pain, and migraines,[39] the studies do not show an independent effect of SSRIs on GI pain.

In summary, SSRIs may help in treating FGIDs because (1) They improve global well-being and some GI-specific symptoms (independent of the effects on depression); (2) They have anxiolytic properties and can target social phobia, agoraphobia, and symptom-related anxiety; (3) They may augment the analgesic effects of other agents (TCAs); and (4) They treat psychiatric comorbidities. In contrast to the dose ranging needed with TCAs, SSRIs do not require much dose readjustment because of selective receptor affinity for 5-HT. Thus, diarrhea may be a side effect, and SSRIs may benefit patients with constipation. Within the SSRI class, paroxetine has more muscarinic effect and may be useful for those with predominant diarrhea. Fluoxetine has a longer half-life and fewer withdrawal effects and may be selected if poor compliance is an issue. Side effects include agitation, hostility, and suicidality.

Serotonin-Norepinephrine Reuptake Inhibitor

A recent study (2008) has evaluated the efficacy of venlafaxine, a serotonin-norepinephrine reuptake inhibitor (SNRI), in patients with functional dyspepsia (FD).[40] The SNRIs, including venlafaxine, duloxetine, and desvenlafaxine, may potentially be as effective as the TCAs, due to their dual blockade of reuptake of NE and 5-HT receptors. Currently, these agents are gaining increased use for other somatic painful conditions such as fibromyalgia.

Duloxetine

Duloxetine is used in chronic pain conditions such as peripheral neuropathy and also pain associated with depression.[41] Benefits may be achieved through its effects on descending 5-HT and NE pain inhibition systems. It lacks activity on muscarinic, histamine, and adrenergic sites, and thus avoids the side effects seen with TCAs. Duloxetine can be started at 30 mg daily and increased up to 60 mg. The most common side effects are nausea, dry mouth, and constipation. Sexual side effects are less common with these agents than with SSRIs. Nonspecific elevation of liver enzymes may also be seen.

Venlafaxine

Venlafaxine inhibits both 5-HT and NE reuptake and can increase stimulated pain threshold.[42] However, higher dosages are needed to achieve pain benefit. It is also a mild inhibitor of dopamine reuptake. It can improve postprandial accommodation of the proximal stomach and may be used for treating FD.[43] However, a recent multicenter RCT showed no difference from placebo in venlafaxine-treated FD patients.[40] It has also been shown to decrease the sensitivity of the colon to rectal distension.[43] Nausea is a side effect to consider. It can be started at 37.5 mg or 75 mg and titrated up to achieve maximum effect.

Table 3
Recent studies on the use of SSRIs in FGIDs

Citation	Drug	Sample	Study Design	Outcome
Creed et al, 2003[73]	Paroxetine	Severe IBS (n = 257)	3 mo Multicenter parallel RCT	1. Improved physical component of SF-36 (QOL) scale. 2. Decreased health care costs at 1 y follow-up. 3. Decreased severity and number of days in pain.
Kuiken et al, 2003[86]	Fluoxetine	IBS (n = 40)	6 wk Double-blind placebo controlled RCT	1. Improved abdominal pain score (53% vs 26%) showing trends toward significance. 2. Patients on fluoxetine were more likely to continue with the drug (84% vs 37%). 3. Significant reduction in abdominal pain in patients with gut hypersensitivity.
Tabas et al, 2004[87]	Paroxetine	IBS (n = 110)	12 wk Double-blind placebo-controlled RCT	1. Improved overall well-being. 2. Increased desire to continue medication. 3. Less IBS-related anxiety. 4. Decreased food avoidance. 5. Benefit seen in nondepressed patients
Vahedi et al, 2005[88]	Fluoxetine	IBS-C (n = 44)	12 weeks Double-blind RCT	1. Decreased abdominal discomfort and bloating. 2. Increased frequency of bowel movements and decreased stool consistency. 3. Insignificant reduction in the mean number of symptoms per patient.
Tack et al, 2006[8]	Citalopram	IBS patients (n = 23)	6 weeks Double-blind placebo-controlled RCT	1. Improved abdominal pain and bloating. 2. Less impact of symptoms on daily life and improved overall well-being. 3. Effects independent of psychological and colonic sensorimotor function.
Talley et al, 2008[89]	Imipramine and Citalopram	IBS patients (n = 51)	12 wk Multicenter double-blind parallel group RCT	1. Imipramine improved bowel symptom severity rating for interference and distress. 2. Imipramine improved depression and SF-36 (mental component) score. 3. Neither imipramine nor citalopram significantly improved Rome III global IBS endpoint (adequate relief).

Abbreviations: FGIDs, functional gastrointestinal disorders; IBS, irritable bowel syndrome; QOL, quality of life; RCT, randomized controlled trial; SF-36, short-form 36-item questionnaire; SSRIs, selective serotonin reuptake inhibitors.

Desvenlafaxine

Desvenlafaxine is related to venlafaxine in molecular structure and has recently been released for the treatment of depression. Its benefit in painful GI conditions has not yet been studied.

Atypical Antipsychotics

Atypical antipsychotics have gained wide acceptance for the treatment of bipolar disorder and schizophrenia because of their efficacy and low toxicity. They can also be beneficial in lower dosages for patients with FGIDs because of their analgesic properties (alone or in synergism with antidepressants)[44] and their sedative and anxiolytic effects. They can enhance a more normal sleep architecture.[45] In the last three years, we used a low-dose atypical antipsychotic agent (eg, quetiapine 25–100 mg) with dopaminergic actions for augmenting treatment in patients with FGIDs. Preliminary data from our clinic show that about 50% of patients with severe IBS and functional abdominal pain syndrome, who previously failed antidepressants and who are prescribed quetiapine with an antidepressant, stay on it, and most of them do achieve some benefit (M. Grover, MD, unpublished data, 2009). Finally, data are emerging from other medical diseases to show the benefit of this class of drugs for functional visceral and somatic symptoms. Olanzapine has shown promise for treating nausea and vomiting in cancer patients,[46] and quetiapine has shown benefit in the treatment of fibromyalgia,[47] which is commonly associated with IBS.[48] Several of these disorders have hypersensitivity of 5-HT2 receptors, excessive substance P, and NMDA receptor activation, all of which increase the depolarization of second-order neurons carrying sensory input, including pain, to the brain.[49]

Miscellaneous Agents

Mirtazapine

Mirtazapine is a tetracyclic 5-HT and NE drug, acting antagonistically at presynaptic alpha-2 receptors in the CNS. It also has 5-HT2, 5-HT3, and H1 antagonistic and a moderate peripheral alpha-1 adrenergic and anticholinergic action. There have been preliminary reports of its effectiveness in FGIDs.[50] It can be useful in patients with nausea and poor appetite, insomnia, weight loss, and diarrhea. It is effective in nausea because of 5-HT3 antagonistic action.[51] Weight gain is an observed side effect, and it is a preferred agent in patients with anorexia.

Buspirone

Buspirone is an anxiolytic used alone or in combination with SSRIs or TCAs. It acts via non-benzodiazepine γ-aminobutyric acid receptors. It has strong affinity for 5-HT1 and 5-HT2 receptors and moderate affinity for D2 receptors. Buspirone can be used in FD to increase receptive relaxation or as noted to augment therapy (see below) with other antidepressants.[52] Its action on 5-HT1 receptor produces relaxation of gastric fundus and improves gastric compliance.[43] The effect on colonic tone has been inconsistent.[43]

Benzodiazepines

Despite the fact that benzodiazepines (BZDs) and barbiturates (Butibel or Donnatal) are often prescribed in FGIDs, there is only limited anecdotal evidence that these agents may have a possible beneficial effect in IBS patients with anxiety disorders.[53] The addiction potential, worsening of associated depression, and poor safety profile of these agents make them less-attractive candidates.

Combination/Augmentation Therapy

Within psychiatry, combinations of two psychopharmacologic agents with different mechanisms of action used at low doses have been used to augment efficacy and minimize side effects. This strategy can be particularly helpful if patients are unable to tolerate higher doses of an agent due to side effects or if they have severe and refractory symptoms that have not been responsive to usual treatments, for example, with a single antidepressant. In general, both buspirone and bupropion have been successfully used as augmentation agents for the treatment of depression.[52]

In our clinical experience, buspirone, a non-benzodiazepine azapirone with anti-anxiety properties, has been shown to enhance the analgesic effect of antidepressants. It can also be prescribed in patients with non-ulcer dyspepsia or chronic nausea because of its effects on gastric relaxation. In addition, our experience with the atypical antipsychotic quetiapine to augment therapy with antidepressants confirms that a combination of low doses of two different classes of agents is worth investigation in the therapy of FGIDs. A low-dose BZD initially combined with an SSRI is an effective strategy in patients with panic disorder, though it is more desirable eventually for the BZD to be reduced or discontinued over time. SSRIs can be added to low-dose TCAs to possibly enhance an analgesic effect, but it is particularly helpful to augment the treatment of psychiatric comorbidities, such as anxiety and depressive disorders as well as panic, generalized social phobia, and obsessive-compulsive disorder. Agitation and delusional symptoms are amenable to atypical antipsychotics or a mental health referral. Managing side effects while being on one of these agents is prudent to ensure compliance. Therefore, this approach of combining two different classes of drugs requires knowledge of the therapeutic class of drug and the effect desired, and it may require a psychiatric referral for initial planning and maintenance of augmentation therapy.

BEHAVIORAL TREATMENTS
General Approach

Behavioral treatments have advantages because of their safety and ability to target factors contributing to symptom perpetuation. These include modifying maladaptive illness beliefs (such as "I can never get better," "My symptoms will lead to cancer," etc), behaviors (such as fear-based avoidance and withdrawal from activities) called "catastrophizing," symptom-specific anxiety (specific fears about symptoms and activities associated with symptoms), and feelings of helplessness and lack of control. Although treatments such as cognitive behavior therapy (CBT), brief psychodynamic therapy, and hypnosis differ in their theoretic underpinnings and the content of what transpires during the sessions, they address the same issue (albeit with differences in emphasis on specific targets). No one treatment is superior to the other, and decision is based on the availability and skill of the therapist and the interests of the patient.[54] Referral to a behavioral therapist is advised based on symptom severity, presence of maladaptive coping, and when the patient sees a relation of stress with symptoms and is motivated toward treatment. Predictors of favorable treatment response are confidence in treatment success, perceived sense of control over the symptoms, and a good relationship with the therapist.[55] These behavioral treatments can be synergistic to medical treatments. Furthermore, there are no side effects, benefits are beyond the end of treatment, and they have been shown to reduce health care costs.

Cognitive Behavior Therapy

CBT is based on social learning theory, which recognizes that behavior is shaped as a result of its social consequences. It focuses on ways to increase or decrease thoughts and behaviors. In the treatment of FGIDs, it typically consists of 3 components: cognitive change where patients learn to recognize the relationship between their beliefs and symptoms, addressing thoughts, behaviors, and responses that result from their experiences, and changing behavior by teaching relaxation and stress management strategies. The specific content of the therapy is based on a biopsychosocial assessment of the patient's background and current difficulties. For example, if a history of sexual abuse interferes with adaptation to the disorder, factors related to the abuse will be discussed. Similarly, if family, job, or other environmental factors related to symptom flare-ups occur, they too will be addressed. Some studies showed that CBT leads to greater reduction in GI symptoms compared with that with symptom monitoring or self-help support group,[56,57] and this may be more efficient when using group formats.[58,59] In a large study, CBT was found to be more effective than educational intervention in terms of symptom relief and global well-being after 3 months, but with minimal effect on pain scores or HRQOL. There was improved coping, and the effects were independent of severity of symptoms, or whether there was a history of abuse or depression, but showed less benefit for patients with higher depression scores.[7] In other studies, specially trained nurses provided effective CBT to IBS patients in primary care, and these effects persisted for up to 6 months.[60] Symptom benefit with CBT may be mediated through changes in the neural activity of cortical-limbic regions that subserve hypervigilance and emotion regulation.[61] It has also been shown that CBT has a direct effect on global IBS symptom improvement independent of its effects on distress; however, there was improvement in the QOL, which may lower distress.[62] In a study in 2008, a brief patient-administered CBT regimen was capable of providing short-term relief from refractory IBS symptoms.[63] To date, when considering the most methodologically strong studies, CBT has been proven to be an effective psychotherapy for treatment of FGIDs.

Relaxation Training

Relaxation techniques are to train patients to counteract the physiologic sequelae of stress or anxiety. Relaxation alone[64] or in combination with CBT and other therapies[65] has been shown to be beneficial in targeting IBS symptoms. One study has shown it to be as effective in reducing GI symptoms as combined relaxation and CBT.[66]

Combined Psychotherapies

Several studies have shown that combined muscle relaxation training with CBT is superior to waiting list controls or conventional therapy.[67] Benefits of this combination compared with those of active education control have yielded mixed results. Relaxation training combined with psychodrama was no better than standard therapy for GI symptoms but had greater anxiolytic effects.[68] The combination of medical treatment plus multicomponent behavioral treatment has been shown to be superior to medical treatment alone in the therapy of IBS.[69]

Dynamic Interpersonal Psychotherapy

Psychodynamic interpersonal therapy (PIT) focuses on the impact of GI symptoms on a person's feelings and relationships. Unlike CBT, the emphasis is on addressing the person's feelings and inner mood states as they relate to flare-ups of symptoms rather than modifying thoughts or cognitions. Bowel disorders affect relationships and family life in a way that can become counterproductive and even damaging for the person with bowel problems and his/her family. PIT looks at the whole marital/relationship system or family system where appropriate, and it can help address and manage issues related to previous sexual/physical abuse. Problems or difficulties with emotions or relationships are brought alive in the sessions and possible solutions tried and tested out with the therapist, before transference to real-life situations. At the end of the therapy, the patient is provided with a detailed personal letter outlining the key points of therapy, plans for the future, and ways to cope with bowel symptoms should they recur.[70] The key to success is the development of a trusting and supportive relationship with the treating therapist. PIT has been used with success in the treatment of refractory FGIDs by Guthrie and colleagues, who reported improvement in symptoms, lesser disability, and lesser health care use.[71,72] Creed and colleagues when comparing usual medical treatment to paroxetine and PIT found that paroxetine and PIT significantly reduced pain scores and improved HRQOL compared with the usual medical treatment. However, only the psychotherapy group had a reduction in health care cost in the 1-year follow-up period. This study is the first to show that SSRIs may play a role in the treatment of FGIDs and that patients with a history of sexual abuse can do particularly well.[73]

Hypnotherapy

The essence of hypnotherapy is to create a relaxing, calming environment that allows the patients to refocus away from their uncomfortable symptoms and toward a more pleasant perception of their current state. It capitalizes on the use of heightened suggestibility where the patients become receptive to viewing their symptoms in a more refocused and positive way. Hypnotherapy has been shown to be effective for the treatment of IBS,[74] and a recent review concluded that hypnosis has a favorable impact on refractory IBS symptoms.[75] One approach directs the patient away from experiencing uncomfortable sensations, such as pain, toward more positive interpretations of the sensations, such as a gentle "flowing" of their bowels. Its long-term efficacy in IBS[76] and FD[77] has been shown. Thus, hypnotherapy is becoming increasingly recognized as a viable treatment modality for IBS.[76–78] The mechanism is unclear, though there is some evidence that it reduces gut contractility and aids in normalization of pain thresholds after balloon rectal distension,[12] though this has not been confirmed by other investigators.[79] Some researchers have demonstrated changes similar to those after CBT,[11] with reduction in anxiety and somatization scores[79] without physiologic changes in the gut.

Mindfulness Meditation

Compared with relaxation, which is a passive state of mind, mindfulness meditation is an active, yet relaxed, state of consciousness. Initial pilot studies have shown promising results for chronic medical and psychiatric conditions. Relaxation response meditation showed significant improvement in flatulence and belching compared with controls.[80]

Limitations of Behavioral Treatments

Behavioral treatments require considerable patient motivation. Patients need to understand and accept the plan and be available for frequent visits with the therapist. This may be costly, because currently, there is poor reimbursement from third-party payers, though in the long term, psychological treatment is more cost effective than medical treatments.[73] It also requires a trained therapist in the community who has experience in working with GI disorders.

COMBINED PSYCHOPHARMACOLOGIC AND BEHAVIORAL TREATMENTS

Fig 1 offers an algorithmic approach to the treatment of FGIDs from mild to severe, once the diagnosis is established. For the majority of patients with mild symptoms, symptomatic medical treatment (mostly gut acting agents) is warranted. Psychotropic drugs and/or psychotherapy are usually initiated with more moderate and persistent symptoms. Generally, a low-dose TCA or another antidepressant can be tried, and if the patient is motivated, psychological intervention can be considered. As the symptoms become more severe and there is higher functional limitation and increased psychological distress, combination therapies (2 psychotropic drugs or psychotropic drugs and behavioral treatments) are required. The figure also provides "red flags" to help the clinician decide when in particular psychological intervention is needed.

The rationale for combined treatments relate to differential effects of antidepressants as related to behavioral treatments that are complementary. Antidepressants improve pain, vegetative signs, and hopelessness and can improve motivation for psychological treatment. Psychological treatments improve coping, cognitive functioning, and effects of trauma and increase adherence to medication. Brain imaging shows that antidepressants have a bottom-up effect acting on paralimbic (cingulate, insula), and psychological treatments have top-down effects acting on prefrontal cognitive areas and improving executive functioning. Based on the literature in IBS, these treatments may not improve the pain as much as the patient's adaptation to the pain and increased coping strategies. In implementing psychological treatment, it is critical that the referring physician help the patients accept the value of these treatments as part of their ongoing care plan.

SUMMARY

With the evolving understanding of the etiopathogenesis and clinical manifestations of FGIDs, the use of centrally acting psychopharmacologic and behavioral treatments is expected to grow. There is evidence for the role of psychosocial factors on FGID disease processes and treatment outcomes. Although better-designed treatment trials are needed, the existing evidence favors the use of both psychopharmacologic and behavioral therapies. To enhance the therapeutic effect and improve adherence to treatment, an effective physician–patient relationship is essential, and guidelines for this can be found elsewhere.[81,82] Future work in the management of FGIDs will lead to the evaluation of multicomponent treatments (eg, the common combination of psychotherapy and pharmacotherapy) and physician treatment behaviors.

REFERENCES

1. Drossman DA, Corazziari E, Delvaux M, et al. Rome III: the functional gastrointestinal disorders. 3rd edition. McLean (VA): Degnon Associates; 2006.
2. Spiller R. Recent advances in understanding the role of serotonin in gastrointestinal motility in functional bowel disorders: alterations in 5-HT signalling and metabolism in human disease. Neurogastroenterol Motil 2007;19(Suppl 2):25–31.
3. Mayer EA, Naliboff BD, Craig AD. Neuroimaging of the brain-gut axis: from basic understanding to treatment of functional GI disorders. Gastroenterology 2006; 131:1925–42.
4. Mayer EA, Tillisch K, Bradesi S. Review article: modulation of the brain-gut axis as a therapeutic approach in gastrointestinal disease. Aliment Pharmacol Ther 2006; 24:919–33.

5. Clouse RE, Lustman PJ. Use of psychopharmacological agents for functional gastrointestinal disorders. Gut 2005;54:1332–41.
6. Lesbros-Pantoflickova D, Michetti P, Fried M, et al. Meta-analysis: the treatment of irritable bowel syndrome. Aliment Pharmacol Ther 2004;20:1253–69.
7. Drossman DA, Toner BB, Whitehead WE, et al. Cognitive-behavioral therapy versus education and desipramine versus placebo for moderate to severe functional bowel disorders. Gastroenterology 2003;125:19–31.
8. Tack J, Broekaert D, Fischler B, et al. A controlled crossover study of the selective serotonin reuptake inhibitor citalopram in irritable bowel syndrome. Gut 2006;55:1095–103.
9. Gorard DA, Libby GW, Farthing MJ. Influence of antidepressants on whole gut and orocaecal transit times in health and irritable bowel syndrome. Aliment Pharmacol Ther 1994;8:159–66.
10. Creed F, Guthrie E, Ratcliffe J, et al. Does psychological treatment help only those patients with severe irritable bowel syndrome who also have a concurrent psychiatric disorder? Aust N Z J Psychiatry 2005;39:807–15.
11. Gonsalkorale WM, Toner BB, Whorwell PJ. Cognitive change in patients undergoing hypnotherapy for irritable bowel syndrome. J Psychosom Res 2004;56:271–8.
12. Lea R, Houghton LA, Calvert EL, et al. Gut-focused hypnotherapy normalizes disordered rectal sensitivity in patients with irritable bowel syndrome. Aliment Pharmacol Ther 2003;17:635–42.
13. Spanier JA, Howden CW, Jones MP. A systematic review of alternative therapies in the irritable bowel syndrome. Arch Intern Med 2003;163:265–74.
14. Talley NJ, Owen BK, Boyce P, et al. Psychological treatments for irritable bowel syndrome: a critique of controlled treatment trials. Am J Gastroenterol 1996;91:277–83.
15. Lydiard RB. Irritable bowel syndrome, anxiety, and depression: what are the links? J Clin Psychiatry 2001;62(Suppl 8):38–45.
16. Drossman DA. The functional gastrointestinal disorders and the Rome III process. Gastroenterology 2006;130:1377–90.
17. Drossman DA, Talley NJ, Olden KW, et al. Sexual and physical abuse and gastrointestinal illness: review and recommendations. Ann Intern Med 1995;123:782–94.
18. Drossman DA, Li Z, Leserman J, et al. Health status by gastrointestinal diagnosis and abuse history. Gastroenterology 1996;110:999–1007.
19. Drossman DA, Whitehead WE, Toner BB, et al. What determines severity among patients with painful functional bowel disorders? Am J Gastroenterol 2000;95:974–80.
20. Posserud I, Agerforz P, Ekman R, et al. Altered visceral perceptual and neuroendocrine response in patients with irritable bowel syndrome during mental stress. Gut 2004;53:1102–8.
21. Drossman DA. Mind over matter in the postinfective irritable bowel. Gut 1999;44:306–7.
22. North CS, Downs D, Clouse RE, et al. The presentation of irritable bowel syndrome in the context of somatization disorder. Clin Gastroenterol Hepatol 2004;2:787–95.
23. Drossman DA. Brain imaging and its implications for studying centrally targeted treatments in IBS: a primer for gastroenterologists. Gut 2005;54:569–73.
24. Mayeux R, Drossman DA, Basham KK, et al. Gulf war and health: physiologic, psychologic, and psychosocial effects of deployment-related stress. Washington, DC: The National Academies Press; 2007.

25. North CS, Hong BA, Alpers DH. Relationship of functional gastrointestinal disorders and psychiatric disorders: implications for treatment. World J Gastroenterol 2007;13:2020–7.
26. Thiwan SM, Drossman DA. Treatment of functional GI disorders with psychotropic medicines: a review of evidence with a practical approach. Gastroenterology & Hepatology 2006;2:678–88.
27. Prakash C, Clouse RE. Long-term outcome from tricyclic antidepressant treatment of functional chest pain. Dig Dis Sci 1999;44:2373–9.
28. Mertz HR. Irritable bowel syndrome. N Engl J Med 2003;349:2136–46.
29. Sayuk GS, Elwing JE, Lustman PJ, et al. Predictors of premature antidepressant discontinuation in functional gastrointestinal disorders. Psychosom Med 2007;69: 173–81.
30. Clouse RE, Lustman PJ, Geisman RA, et al. Antidepressant therapy in 138 patients with irritable bowel syndrome: a five-year clinical experience. Aliment Pharmacol Ther 1994;8:409–16.
31. Bomholt SF, Mikkelsen JD, Blackburn-Munro G. Antinociceptive effects of the antidepressants amitriptyline, duloxetine, mirtazapine and citalopram in animal models of acute, persistent and neuropathic pain. Neuropharmacology 2005; 48:252–63.
32. Su X, Gebhart GF. Effects of tricyclic antidepressants on mechanosensitive pelvic nerve afferent fibers innervating the rat colon. Pain 1998;76:105–14.
33. Willert RP, Woolf CJ, Hobson AR, et al. The development and maintenance of human visceral pain hypersensitivity is dependent on the N-methyl-D-aspartate receptor. Gastroenterology 2004;126:683–92.
34. Gorelick AB, Koshy SS, Hooper FG, et al. Differential effects of amitriptyline on perception of somatic and visceral stimulation in healthy humans. Am J Phys 1998;275:G460–6.
35. Choung RS, Cremonini F, Thapa P, et al. The effect of short-term, low-dose tricyclic and tetracyclic antidepressant treatment on satiation, postnutrient load gastrointestinal symptoms and gastric emptying: a double-blind, randomized, placebo-controlled trial. Neurogastroenterol Motil 2008;20:220–7.
36. Drossman DA, Ringel Y, Vogt BA, et al. Alterations of brain activity associated with resolution of emotional distress and pain in a case of severe irritable bowel syndrome. Gastroenterology 2003;124:754–61.
37. Ringel Y, Drossman DA, Leserman JL, et al. Effect of abuse history on pain reports and brain responses to aversive visceral stimulation: an FMRI study. Gastroenterology 2008;134:396–404.
38. Morgan V, Pickens D, Gautam S, et al. Amitriptyline reduces rectal pain related activation of the anterior cingulate cortex in patients with irritable bowel syndrome. Gut 2005;54:601–7.
39. Creed F. How do SSRIs help patients with irritable bowel syndrome? Gut 2006;55: 1065–7.
40. van Kerkhoven LA, Laheij RJ, Aparicio N, et al. Effect of the antidepressant venlafaxine in functional dyspepsia: a randomized, double-blind, placebo-controlled trial. Clin Gastroenterol Hepatol 2008;6:746–52.
41. Brannan SK, Mallinckrodt CH, Brown EB, et al. Duloxetine 60 mg once-daily in the treatment of painful physical symptoms in patients with major depressive disorder. J Psychiatr Res 2005;39:43–53.
42. Bradley RH, Barkin RL, Jerome J, et al. Efficacy of venlafaxine for the long term treatment of chronic pain with associated major depressive disorder. Am J Ther 2003;10:318–23.

43. Chial HJ, Camilleri M, Ferber I, et al. Effects of venlafaxine, buspirone, and placebo on colonic sensorimotor functions in healthy humans. Clin Gastroenterol Hepatol 2003;1:211–8.

44. Fishbain DA, Cutler RB, Lewis J, et al. Do the second-generation "atypical neuroleptics" have analgesic properties? A structured evidence-based review. Pain Med 2004;5:359–65.

45. Hamner MB, Deitsch SE, Brodrick PS, et al. Quetiapine treatment in patients with posttraumatic stress disorder: an open trial of adjunctive therapy. J Clin Psychopharmacol 2003;23:15–20.

46. Passik SD, Lundberg J, Kirsh KL, et al. A pilot exploration of the antiemetic activity of olanzapine for the relief of nausea in patients with advanced cancer and pain. J Pain Symptom Manage 2002;23:526–32.

47. Hidalgo J, Rico-Villademoros F, Calandre EP. An open-label study of quetiapine in the treatment of fibromyalgia. Prog Neuropsychopharmacol Biol Psychiatry 2007;31:71–7.

48. Pimentel M, Wallace D, Hallegua D, et al. A link between irritable bowel syndrome and fibromyalgia may be related to findings on lactulose breath testing. Ann Rheum Dis 2004;63:450–2.

49. Smith NL. Serotonin mechanisms in pain and functional syndromes: management implications in comorbid fibromyalgia, headache, and irritable bowl syndrome—case study and discussion. J Pain Palliat Care Pharmacother 2004;18:31–45.

50. Thomas SG. Irritable bowel syndrome and mirtazapine. Am J Psychiatry 2000;157:1341–2.

51. Thompson DS. Mirtazapine for the treatment of depression and nausea in breast and gynecological oncology. Psychosomatics 2000;41:356–9.

52. Trivedi MH, Fava M, Wisniewski SR, et al. Medication augmentation after the failure of SSRIs for depression. N Engl J Med 2006;354:1243–52.

53. Tollefson GD, Luxenberg M, Valentine R, et al. An open label trial of alprazolam in comorbid irritable bowel syndrome and generalized anxiety disorder. J Clin Psychiatry 1991;52:502–8.

54. Creed F, Levy R, Bradley L, et al. Psychosocial aspects of functional gastrointestinal disorders. In: Drossman DA, Corazziari E, Delvaux M, et al, editors. Rome III: the functional gastrointestinal disorders. 3rd edition. McLean (VA): Degnon Associates; 2006. p. 295–368.

55. Drossman DA, Toner BB, Morris CB, et al. What characterizes a response to cognitive-behavioral treatment in a functional bowel clinical trial? Gastroenterology 2005;128(4 Suppl 2):A66.

56. Payne A, Blanchard EB. A controlled comparison of cognitive therapy and self-help support groups in the treatment of irritable bowel syndrome. J Consult Clin Psychol 1995;63:779–86.

57. Greene B, Blanchard EB. Cognitive therapy for irritable bowel syndrome. J Consult Clin Psychol 1994;62:576–82.

58. Toner BB, Segal ZV, Emmott S, et al. Cognitive-behavioral group therapy for patients with irritable bowel syndrome. Int J Group Psychother 1998;48:215–43.

59. Blanchard EB, Lackner JM, Sanders K, et al. A controlled evaluation of group cognitive therapy in the treatment of irritable bowel syndrome. Behav Res Ther 2007;45:633–48.

60. Kennedy TM, Chalder T, McCrone P, et al. Cognitive behavioural therapy in addition to antispasmodic therapy for irritable bowel syndrome in primary care: randomised controlled trial. Health Technol Assess 2006;10:iii–x.

61. Lackner JM, Lou CM, Mertz HR, et al. Cognitive therapy for irritable bowel syndrome is associated with reduced limbic activity, GI symptoms, and anxiety. Behav Res Ther 2006;44:621–38.

62. Lackner JM, Jaccard J, Krasner SS, et al. How does cognitive behavior therapy for irritable bowel syndrome work? A mediational analysis of a randomized clinical trial. Gastroenterology 2007;133:433–44.

63. Lackner JM, Jaccard J, Krasner SS, et al. Self-administered cognitive behavior therapy for moderate to severe irritable bowel syndrome: clinical efficacy, tolerability, feasibility. Clin Gastroenterol Hepatol 2008;6:899–906.

64. Voirol MW, Hipolito J. [Anthropo-analytical relaxation in irritable bowel syndrome: results 40 months later]. Schweiz Med Wochenschr 1987;117:1117–9 [English].

65. Blanchard EB, Schwarz SP, Suls JM, et al. Two controlled evaluations of multicomponent psychological treatment of irritable bowel syndrome. Behav Res Ther 1992;30:175–89.

66. Blanchard EB, Greene B, Scharff L, et al. Relaxation training as a treatment for irritable bowel syndrome. Biofeedback Self Regul 1993;18:125–32.

67. Drossman DA, Creed F, Olden KW, et al. Psychosocial aspects of functional gastrointestinal disorders. In: Drossman DA, Corazziari E, Talley NJ, et al, editors. Rome II: the functional gastrointestinal disorders. 2nd edition. McLean (VA): Degnon Associates; 2000. p. 157–245.

68. Arn I, Theorell T, Uvnas-Moberg K, et al. Psychodrama group therapy for patients with functional gastrointestinal disorders—a controlled long-term follow-up study. Psychother Psychosom 1989;51:113–9.

69. Heymann-Monnikes I, Arnold R, Florin I, et al. The combination of medical treatment plus multicomponent behavioral therapy is superior to medical treatment alone in the therapy of irritable bowel syndrome. Am J Gastroenterol 2000;95:981–94.

70. Howlett S, Guthrie E. Use of farewell letters in the context of brief psychodynamic-interpersonal therapy with irritable bowel syndrome patients. British Journal of Psychotherapy 2001;18(1):52–67.

71. Guthrie E, Creed F, Dawson D, et al. A controlled trial of psychological treatment for the irritable bowel syndrome. Gastroenterology 1991;100:450–7.

72. Hamilton J, Guthrie E, Creed F, et al. A randomized controlled trial of psychotherapy in patients with chronic functional dyspepsia. Gastroenterology 2000;119:661–9.

73. Creed F, Fernandes L, Guthrie E, et al. The cost-effectiveness of psychotherapy and paroxetine for severe irritable bowel syndrome. Gastroenterology 2003;124:303–17.

74. Whorwell PJ, Prior A, Faragher EB. Controlled trial of hypnotherapy in the treatment of severe refractory irritable-bowel syndrome. Lancet 1984;2:1232–4.

75. Whitehead WE. Hypnosis for irritable bowel syndrome: the empirical evidence of therapeutic effects. Int J Clin Exp Hypn 2006;54:7–20.

76. Gonsalkorale WM, Miller V, Afzal A, et al. Long term benefits of hypnotherapy for irritable bowel syndrome. Gut 2003;52:1623–9.

77. Calvert EL, Houghton LA, Cooper P, et al. Long-term improvement in functional dyspepsia using hypnotherapy. Gastroenterology 2002;123:1778–85.

78. Gonsalkorale WM, Houghton LA, Whorwell PJ. Hypnotherapy in irritable bowel syndrome: a large-scale audit of a clinical service with examination of factors influencing responsiveness. Am J Gastroenterol 2002;97:954–61.

79. Palsson OS, Turner MJ, Johnson DA, et al. Hypnosis treatment for severe irritable bowel syndrome: investigation of mechanism and effects on symptoms. Dig Dis Sci 2002;47:2605–14.

80. Keefer L, Blanchard EB. The effects of relaxation response meditation on the symptoms of irritable bowel syndrome: results of a controlled treatment study. Behav Res Ther 2001;39:801–11.

81. Chang L, Drossman DA. Optimizing patient care: the psychosocial interview in the irritable bowel syndrome. Clinical perspectives in gastroenterology 2002;5: 336–41.
82. Halpert A, Dalton CB, Diamant NE, et al. Clinical response to tricyclic antidepressants in functional bowel disorders is not related to dosage. Am J Gastroenterol 2005;100:664–71.
83. Otaka M, Jin M, Odashima M, et al. New strategy of therapy for functional dyspepsia using famotidine, mosapride and amitriptyline. Aliment Pharmacol Ther 2005;21(Suppl 2):42–6.
84. Vahedi H, Merat S, Momtahen S, et al. Clinical trial: the effect of amitriptyline in patients with diarrhoea-predominant irritable bowel syndrome. Aliment Pharmacol Ther 2008;27:678–84.
85. Bahar RJ, Collins BS, Steinmetz B, et al. Double-blind placebo-controlled trial of amitriptyline for the treatment of irritable bowel syndrome in adolescents. J Pediatr 2008;152:685–9.
86. Kuiken SD, Tytgat GN, Boeckxstaens GE. The selective serotonin reuptake inhibitor fluoxetine does not change rectal sensitivity and symptoms in patients with irritable bowel syndrome: a double blind, randomized, placebo-controlled study. Clin Gastroenterol Hepatol 2003;1:219–28.
87. Tabas G, Beaves M, Wang J, et al. Paroxetine to treat irritable bowel syndrome not responding to high-fiber diet: a double-blind, placebo-controlled trial. Am J Gastroenterol 2004;99:914–20.
88. Vahedi H, Merat S, Rashidioon A, et al. The effect of fluoxetine in patients with pain and constipation-predominant irritable bowel syndrome: a double-blind randomized-controlled study. Aliment Pharmacol Ther 2005;22:381–5.
89. Talley NJ, Kellow JE, Boyce P, et al. Antidepressant therapy (imipramine and citalopram) for irritable bowel syndrome: a double-blind, randomized, placebo-controlled trial. Dig Dis Sci 2008;53:108–15.

The Gastrointestinal Motility Laboratory

Henry P. Parkman, MD[a],*, William C. Orr, PhD[b]

KEYWORDS

- Motility testing • Esophageal manometry
- Esophageal pH recording • Anal manometry

Gastrointestinal (GI) motility and functional GI disorders are common and often perplexing problems encountered by the gastroenterologist (**Table 1**). GI and functional GI disorders affect up to 25% of the American population,[1] comprise about 40% of GI problems for which patients seek health care,[2] and are common reasons for patients to see gastroenterologists. For the patients, they cause symptoms and pose a heavy burden of illness, decreasing quality of life and work productivity.[3–5] Proper evaluation of these disorders is important to care for these patients appropriately in clinical practice.

The GI motility laboratory can provide useful, if not definitive, information about the diagnosis and management of some of the most common problems confronted by gastroenterologists. These include heartburn, dysphagia, chest pain, chronic cough, chronic constipation, and fecal incontinence. Less common disorders, such as achalasia and scleroderma, have esophageal motor abnormalities that can also be diagnosed and managed more effectively by way of esophageal motility and 24-hour esophageal pH studies.

Proper evaluation of patients who have suspected GI motility disorders is important to diagnose the patient's condition correctly and to treat the patient in an appropriate manner. Tests of GI motility allow the assessment and identification of abnormal patterns and physiology. Symptom-based definitions are often used to make a positive diagnosis for functional bowel disorders.[6] A GI motility procedure is often used for further evaluation to detect some specific physiologic dysfunction.[7] Usually, these procedures are performed after upper endoscopy or colonoscopy is performed to rule out an obstructive lesion. For instance, for esophageal symptoms, esophageal manometry and esophageal pH monitoring are used to determine the presence of gastroesophageal reflux disease (GERD) and to assess esophageal motor function.

This article appeared previously in the September 2007 issue of Gastroenterology Clinics of North America (36:3), with permission.

[a] Gastroenterology Section, Department of Medicine, Temple University School of Medicine, Parkinson Pavilion, 8th Floor, 3401 North Broad Street, Philadelphia, PA 19140, USA

[b] Lynn Health Science Institute, University of Oklahoma Health Sciences Center, 5300 N. Independence, Suite 130, Oklahoma City, OK 73112, USA

* Corresponding author.

E-mail address: henry.parkman@temple.edu (H.P. Parkman).

Table 1
An anatomic classification of gastrointestinal motility and functional gastrointestinal disorders

Organ	GI Motility Disorders	Functional GI Disorders
Esophagus	Achalasia	Functional dysphagia
	Diffuse esophageal spasm	Functional chest pain
	Gastroesophageal reflux disease	Functional heartburn
Stomach	Gastroparesis	Functional dyspepsia
	Dumping syndrome	Cyclic vomiting syndrome
Small intestine	Chronic intestinal pseudoobstruction	Irritable bowel syndrome
	Small intestinal bacterial overgrowth	
Biliary tract	Gallbladder hypomotility	
	Sphincter of Oddi dysfunction	
Colon	Colonic inertia	Irritable bowel syndrome
	Pelvic floor dyssynergia	Functional constipation
	Hirschsprung's disease	Functional incontinence
		Functional diarrhea

For other symptoms such as heartburn, motility tests are used to evaluate patients who have refractory or atypical symptoms that do not respond to medications.

As the pathogenesis of GI motility disorders and functional bowel disorders becomes better understood, the ability to conduct studies in GI motility becomes increasingly relevant. Motility disorders also play an increasingly recognized role in issues outside of traditional gastroenterology, such as nutrition, obesity, and drug delivery. The ability to measure intestinal motor function in the GI motility laboratory enhances the understanding of abnormal functioning of the luminal GI tract, and also allows the establishment of a relationship between symptoms and identifiable motor abnormalities.

This article addresses important concepts in setting up and running an efficient and practical GI motility laboratory.

GENERAL COMMENTS ON THE GASTROINTESTINAL MOTILITY LABORATORY

The goals of GI motility testing are to allow the assessment of GI physiology and to identify patterns of abnormal physiology, which can provide the correct diagnosis of GI motility disorders, guide the treatment of patients, and provide prognostic information for patients. Some examples of the importance of motility testing in the diagnosis and guidance of treatment are readily apparent in clinical practice. For example, esophageal pH monitoring can evaluate patients for GERD. Esophageal manometry can specifically diagnose achalasia and provide the rationale for effective treatments. Anal manometry can determine if the cause of constipation is dyssynergic defecation or evacuation disorders for which biofeedback may be recommended. Anorectal manometry is also helpful for evaluating fecal incontinence to determine any sensory or motor dysfunction. Advances in technology have greatly improved the ability to measure intestinal motility and to measure these functions in an ambulatory setting, thereby greatly improving the understanding of the relationship between symptoms and motor abnormalities, which, in time, can be better linked by way of prolonged ambulatory monitoring.

Another advantage of having a comprehensive GI motility laboratory is the opportunity to conduct research and study the pathophysiology of various neurogastroenterology and GI motility disorders. For example, it is difficult to investigate the pathogenesis of GERD in any sophisticated manner without the availability of esophageal motility and 24-hour esophageal pH recordings, especially in a patient who has unexplained heartburn or chest pain after a negative endoscopy or failure to respond to proton pump inhibitor therapy. Similarly, the proper study of constipation and its pathophysiology cannot be accomplished without the ability to assess anorectal function. Academic practitioners and research-oriented individuals in clinical practice also have a substantial advantage. By keeping careful records of studies over the years, a rich database can be acquired, which allows research queries to occur that can serve as the basis of a clinical research project. Thus, a GI motility laboratory is an ideal opportunity to meld clinical practice and clinical research.

Unfortunately, experts in GI motility are relatively scarce. It is likely that the comprehensive digestive disease center will have greater access to experts in endoscopic ultrasound than GI motility. Thus, having expertise in GI motility should be a valuable asset as the development of comprehensive digestive centers proliferates. Specialized laboratories in other areas of medicine have been shown recently to be useful and financially feasible, even in smaller hospitals. Perhaps the best example is the development of sleep laboratories. Ten years ago, sleep laboratories were located almost exclusively in academic or tertiary hospitals. With the widespread dissemination of information on the prevalence of sleep disorders, particularly sleep apnea, most hospitals in even smaller communities now have a sleep laboratory. Similarly, the burgeoning of advertising and continuing medical education courses regarding heartburn and acid reflux disease has stimulated the growth of esophageal laboratories not only in hospitals but also in the offices of gastroenterologists.

Based on these observations, it would seem that the GI motility laboratory is poised to grow as the level of diagnostic sophistication in gastroenterology continues to advance. The recent analysis of the future practice of gastroenterology suggests that disorders of GI motility and functional GI disorders will comprise a larger percentage of the GI practice in the future, further increasing the importance of the GI motility laboratory.[8]

THE GASTROINTESTINAL MOTILITY LABORATORY

Several items need to be considered carefully in setting up a practical and efficient GI motility laboratory, including the room, the equipment, the procedures to be performed, the personnel to run the laboratory, billing and coding, and patients.

The Gastrointestinal Motility Laboratory Room

A comprehensive GI laboratory does not require a great deal of space, or even specially configured space. The procedure unit should be readily accessible to inpatients and outpatients.[9] In most centers, the GI motility laboratory is one room, or perhaps two rooms, in the endoscopy suite. This location readily affords easy access to physicians and nurses. Often, the patient may be having endoscopic procedures with manometric procedures, making the GI endoscopy suite location practical. In some instances, the manometric tubes need to be placed with the endoscopic or fluoroscopic guidance.

A few basics are required for the motility room (**Box 1**). The room needs to be a minimum of 14 ft × 16 ft, which should accommodate the necessary equipment and a comfortable bed that can be raised or lowered easily. Ideally, the layout of the

---

Box 1
The gastrointestinal motility laboratory room

Adequate space for conducting tests: 14 × 16 feet

Sink with running water and drain (double basin preferred)

Plenty of electric outlets

Cabinets for storage

Storage rack for catheters

Container for biohazards or sharp disposables

Suction, oxygen

Blood pressure and pulse oximeter machines

Computers and equipment

Desk

Chairs

Telephone

Clock with second hand

Elevatable bed

Crash cart availability

Nearby restroom

Nearby laundry bin

---

room should allow the patient to be accommodated comfortably, and equipment and instruments should be out of view. Electric outlets need to be plentiful. Having the room decorated with some nice landscape pictures is helpful in creating a more comfortable and visually appealing environment. Running water and a large sink are required. A double-basin sink allows cleaning of the equipment and use of running water for other chores. An adequate number of storage cabinets are needed because many supplies, probes, and catheters must be stored. A bed that can be elevated is highly recommended. Suction and oxygen are desirable, but not essential. Bins for regular and biohazard disposable trash must be available in the laboratory space. Near the motility laboratory should be a private bathroom for the patients. An emergency crash cart should be in the vicinity, if not in the actual laboratory space.

Equipment

The equipment for a GI motility laboratory depends on the procedures performed and the types of patients seen in the center (**Box 2**). The comprehensive GI motility laboratory includes the ability to measure luminal GI functioning from mouth to anus. Realistically, however, very few laboratories have a level of comprehensive diagnostic capability that covers this range. Depending on the interest of the specific laboratory director and the types of patients seen, some laboratories may specialize in upper GI motility studies and others in lower GI motility studies (see **Box 2**). However, a GI motility laboratory should have the expertise to perform certain minimum tests, including esophageal manometry, esophageal pH monitoring, and anorectal manometry (**Box 3**). Recently, hydrogen breath testing for bacterial overgrowth and lactose intolerance has become popular. More specialized centers allow referral of patients who may require more sophisticated procedures, such as antroduodenal manometry

---

Box 2
Evaluations in gastrointestinal practice for gastrointestinal motility and functional gastrointestinal disorders

Esophageal symptoms

Esophageal manometry

Esophageal impedance

Esophageal pH monitoring

Esophageal sensory testing with balloon distension

Dyspeptic symptoms

Gastric emptying test

SmartPill pH and pressure capsule

Electrogastrography

Antroduodenal and jejunal manometry

Satiety testing with water or nutrient load

Gastric barostat

Irritable bowel syndrome symptoms

Breath testing

    Bacterial overgrowth

    Lactose intolerance

    Fructose intolerance

Constipation/fecal incontinence

Anal manometry

Anorectal electromyography

Pudendal nerve latency

Balloon expulsion

Colonic transit with sitzmarkers

SmartPill pH and pressure capsule

---

and luminal balloon distention. In the comprehensive digestive disease center, the GI laboratory covers other sophisticated diagnostic services, such as breath testing, capsule endoscopy, and SmartPill transit studies.

Different types and brands of equipment are used for each procedure performed in the GI motility laboratory. Different equipment may perform slightly different tests that assess different functions and provide different types of information (see **Box 3**). The performance characteristics and extent of recording ability of these devices differ and need to be considered, depending on the need of the individual laboratory.[10] For instance, for esophageal manometry, the test can be performed with water-perfused catheters or with solid-state catheters, using conventional spacing of the recording channels or high-resolution systems. In addition, manometry can be combined with impedance to measure esophageal transit and more subtle esophageal motor disorders. For esophageal pH monitoring, one can use a catheter pH probe with one to three pH recording sites, a catheter probe with pH and impedance measurements, or capsule pH monitoring (Bravo pH).

Box 3
Equipment and procedures for the gastrointestinal motility laboratory

First level

Esophageal manometry

Esophageal pH monitoring

Second level

Anal manometry

Balloon expulsion

Anal electromyography

Third level

Breath testing

    Bacterial overgrowth

    Helicobacter pylori

    Lactose intolerance

    Fructose intolerance

Specialized procedures

SmartPill

Antroduodenal manometry

Electrogastrography

Colonic manometry

Barostat studies of stomach and rectum

Biofeedback therapy for constipation and fecal incontinence

Equipment in the laboratory should be Food and Drug Administration–approved with high fidelity. Maintenance of the equipment is important, and cleaning and sterilization between procedures, and regular bioengineering inspection and service, are essential. The laboratory should demonstrate appropriate data acquisition and storage capabilities (archival storage and so forth). The report should include patient data, specific parameters, professional interpretation, and letters to referring physicians. In today's environment of computerized motility studies, data storage is not an issue, but data should be kept for at least 5 years.

Advances in current monitoring techniques allow relatively noninvasive recording of GI motility under physiologic conditions. Novel technologies to evaluate GI motility are being evaluated on a continuing basis. Gastric emptying measurements may shortly enter the GI motility laboratory with the use of SmartPill or breath testing with octanoic acid. Colonic manometry and rectal barostat studies have been added to some laboratories for patient evaluation. Motility laboratories now also function therapeutically, with the performing of anorectal biofeedback for the treatment of constipation and fecal incontinence.

Procedures

Proper performance of GI motility tests is critically important in the evaluation of patients. The Clinical Practice Committee of the American Motility Society has defined standards of practice for a number of clinical motility tests (**Box 4**). These guidelines

---

Box 4
Documents on minimal standards for gastrointestinal motility testing

Esophagus

Murray JA, Clouse RE, Conklin JL. Components of the standard esophageal manometry. Neurogastroent Motil 2003;15(6):591–606.

Stomach

Camilleri M, Hasler W, Parkman HP, et al. Measurement of gastroduodenal motility in the GI laboratory. Gastroenterology 1998;115:747–62.

Parkman HP, Hasler WL, Barnett JL, et al. Electrogastrography: a document prepared by the gastric section of the American Motility Society Clinical GI Motility Testing Task Force. Neurogastroent Motil 2003;75:89–102.

Lin HC, Prather C, Fisher RS, et al. AMS Task Force Committee on Gastrointestinal Transit. Measurement of gastrointestinal transit. Dig Dis Sci 2005;50(6):989–1004.

Colon/rectum

Rao SS, Azpiroz F, Diamant N, et al. Minimum standards of anorectal manometry. Neurogastroent Motil 2002;14(5):553–9.

Biliary tract

Hogan WJ, Sherman S, Pasricha P, et al. Sphincter of Oddi manometry. Gastrointest Endosc 1997;45(3):342–8.

Pediatrics

Di Lorenzo C, Hillemeier C, Hyman P, et al. Manometry studies in children: minimum standards for procedures. Neurogastroent Motil 2002;14(4):411–20.

Billing and coding

Botoman VA, Rao S, Dunlap P, et al. Bill Coding and RVS Committee of the American Motility Society. Motility and GI function studies billing and coding guidelines: a position paper of the American Motility Society. Am J Gastroenterol 2003;98(6):1228–36.

---

help to standardize GI motility procedures better and are useful not only for motility laboratories but also for trainees in learning to appreciate the value of GI motility testing.

Technical and Professional Staff

Director

The director of the laboratory should be an MD or PhD with training and experience in GI motility testing. Because no specific certifications or board examinations certify motility expertise, it must be assessed based on the training and the curriculum vitae of the director. Non-MD professional staff will be expected to have a PhD in one of the related medical sciences (ie, physiology, neurobiology, pharmacology, and so forth).[11] If the director is a PhD, then proper medical oversight must be provided. Expertise in GI motility evaluations should include training in a recognized motility laboratory.

The director of a GI laboratory is most often a gastroenterologist interested in GI motility and functional bowel disorders. Training during gastroenterology fellowship can provide some of the foundation for performing and interpreting GI motility tests.[12] The gastroenterology core curriculum for the training of gastroenterology fellows recommends two training levels in GI motility:[13]

Level 1 Training in GI Motility: Level 1 is basic training in GI motility expected of all GI fellows. GI fellows should understand the pathophysiology of GI motility and functional GI disorders, learn to manage patients with these disorders, and understand the usefulness of the various GI motility tests available to evaluate patients. Trainees should have an appropriate clinical outpatient experience in which to see and manage patients with possible motility disorders. GI fellows should learn about the various GI motility tests including the appropriate indications, interpretation of test results, and appropriate treatment of patients. Trainees should have the opportunity for hands-on experience with GI motility studies, including 24 hour esophageal pH monitoring.

Level 2 Training in GI Motility: Level 2 training is for trainees who wish to have a subspecialty in GI motility and perform motility studies as consultants to other physicians. All directors of GI motility laboratories should have at least this level 2 training. These subspecialty trainees should become familiar with performance and interpretation of a number of different types of GI motility tests. The recommended numbers of studies to achieve expertise was suggested to be 50 esophageal manometry studies, 25 esophageal pH recordings, and 30 anorectal manometry studies. These trainees should also spend at least three months in a GI motility laboratory under the preceptorship of experienced clinicians in the performance of these studies.

The American Neurogastroenterology and Motility Society (ANMS) has developed teaching opportunities for those interested in learning more on GI motility and for those interested in directing a GI motility laboratory.

ANMS course in GI motility: The ANMS gives courses on GI motility in clinical practice for individuals at each level of interest in learning about GI motility (GI fellows, practicing physicians, and nurses/technicians who perform the GI motility procedures). These courses are held every 2 years. The instructors are national experts who are actively practicing in the field of gastrointestinal motility. The goal of these courses is to familiarize participants with, and update them on, the current indications, methodology, and interpretation of clinical GI motility tests. In addition, the courses provide an in-depth and up-to-date discussion of the physiology and pathophysiology and treatment of GI motility and functional bowel disorders.

ANMS clinical training program: Recently, the ANMS has started a clinical training program for fellows and junior faculty in gastrointestinal motility and neurogastroenterology. This program is an apprenticeship-based 1-month training in GI motility and neurogastroenterology for GI fellows and junior faculty in a dedicated GI motility center of excellence. The goal of this training period is to enable participants to learn first hand the various GI motility procedures used to evaluate patients.

Gastrointestinal motility nurse or technician

A dedicated nurse or technician is needed for the GI motility laboratory, to perform the appropriate testing. This person should work full time in the GI motility laboratory. Finding technical staff is challenging. Most nurses and medical assistants have no experience in motility measurements. In most circumstances, staff needs to be trained from scratch. It is advantageous if a nurse can be recruited from the endoscopy laboratory or if he/she has had some GI nursing experience. Specific GI anatomy and disease states will be familiar, making training easier because it can be focused on learning procedures. Training technical staff is largely done in the laboratory as on-the-job training. Some additional training may be obtained from courses sponsored by industry or the ANMS, and these can be very helpful because a great deal of information is concentrated in a short period of time (usually 2 to 3 days). How-ever, the bulk of training is obtained in the local laboratory. Depending on how many procedures are done in the laboratory, effective training of a technician can take between 3 and 6 months.

The involvement of the director varies from laboratory to laboratory. Typically, nurses/technicians can be trained to do the standard laboratory procedures, with the director performing the study interpretation. Some directors have more involve-ment in procedures, depending on the comfort level and particular desires of the director to supervise the conduct of studies. In general, the more involvement and interaction between the director and nurse/technician, the better the clinical care. In most laboratories, the technician conducts all the esophageal studies, whereas a phy-sician and the technician conduct the anorectal procedures together. Typically, stud-ies are interpreted at the end of the day, or the day after the study, and they are sent by fax or mail to the referring physician's office. Constant communication between the laboratory technician and the director is essential. Reviewing tracings and discussing cases should occur on a regular basis to ensure that the technician and director re-main in close agreement on procedure protocol and the recognition of abnormalities that need to be identified during the conduct of the study. An example of this would be proper identification of lower esophageal sphincter pressure and the relaxation of this pressure with swallows, which needs to be recognized on line during a procedure. In patients who have suspected achalasia, it is imperative that this be done properly, which can only be accomplished by constant surveillance of the conduct of the studies by the director, and interaction with the technician.

It is important that the technician be knowledgeable about referrals from different specialists and the specific questions that should be addressed. For example, a refer-ral from a surgeon would need to focus on assessment of peristalsis, especially the magnitude of specific amplitudes of the peristaltic waves, because these may deter-mine how or whether a Nissen fundoplication is done. The technician must be able to recognize that more swallows should be obtained in some circumstances to obtain a reliable assessment of true esophageal function. Similarly, referrals from otolaryn-gologists often dictate a more thorough assessment of the pharynx and upper esoph-ageal sphincter. The technician must communicate effectively with the director about the nature of the referral and any special requests that may have accompanied the specific referral. Referrals for evaluation of rectal pain, as opposed to constipation, may dictate a somewhat different focus on the interpretation by the director and the technician, and director must be knowledgeable about the nature of the referral to perform a proper study and interpretation for the referring physician.

Scheduling coordinator
Different GI motility laboratories handle scheduling differently. Scheduling is usually performed in the office when the patient sees the physician, when the technician is busy performing other GI motility procedures, which often necessitates a medical assistant to schedule the tests. It is important for the scheduling coordinator (eg, med-ical assistant) to understand the essentials of the test (preparation [eg, fasting], med-ications the patient should stop for the test [eg, proton pump inhibitors], the duration of the test, and the order that the test should be performed with others, in case multiple tests are performed the same day).

In some centers, the GI motility technician is involved in scheduling the procedures directly with the patient, or at least in having a conversation with the patient ahead of time, which allows the technician to establish some rapport with the patient and to answer any questions the patient may have concerning the procedure. In addition, the technician can determine and schedule to allow for the most efficient use of time available.

PATIENTS

Patients need to be advised about the preparation for the test and given this in writing. Information should include the preparation for the test (generally fasting after midnight), the need to stop certain medications, and the date, time, and location of the test. Patients also need to understand beforehand what the test will entail. Patient information sheets have been developed for several GI motility procedures (**Box 5**), available through the ANMS website at www.motilitysociety.org. Many patients are apprehensive because, unlike endoscopic procedures, motility studies are usually performed without sedation. Hence, a detailed explanation and repeated reassurance from a compassionate nurse or technician is important for a successful motility laboratory.

Laboratories differ as to whether signed informed consent of patients is needed before performing these tests. Approximately one half of the laboratories have the patient sign an informed consent for the procedure, whereas about one half do not. In general, GI motility tests are low-risk procedures. Esophageal manometry is similar to inserting a nasogastric tube, for which consent is not usually obtained. Others feel that proper informed consent should be obtained for GI motility procedures. Most hospitals have an adequate consent for procedures, which has had appropriate legal review.

Box 5
Patient information sheets on the American Neurogastroenterology and Motility Society website (www.motilitysociety.org)

Gastrointestinal motility tests and procedures

Anal manometry

Esophageal manometry

Esophageal pH monitoring

Gastric emptying scintigraphy

Defecography

Breath hydrogen testing

Small bowel manometry

Gastrointestinal motility disorders

Achalasia

Diffuse esophageal spasm

Chronic intestinal pseudoobstruction

Dumping syndrome diet

Gastroparesis

Gastroparesis diet

Hirschsprung's disease

Useful information on the disorders may be needed for patients who undergo GI motility tests. Patient information has been developed for several GI motility procedures, located and available for downloading on the ANMS web site at www. motilitysociety.org. These can be used for distribution to patients who are undergoing a GI motility procedure.

It is important that a standard format be used for reporting the results of GI motility tests. The ANMS, together with the European Neurogastroenterology and Motility Society, has developed consensus minimum guidelines for testing and reporting of GI motility procedures (see **Box 4**).

BILLING AND CODING

Billing is performed using established *Current Procedural Terminology (CPT)* codes. Virtually all GI motility procedures have codes for the facility fee and interpretation (**Box 6**). Billing and coding are best decided by the individual practitioner, in consultation with respective payers in his/her location.[14]

The ANMS, with the American Gastroenterology Association, American Society for Gastrointestinal Endoscopy, and American College of Gastroenterology, has been striving for improved coding and reimbursement for procedures performed in the GI motility laboratory. Proper reimbursement and constant monitoring of payments is necessary to ensure maximal reimbursement. Insurance companies vary significantly with regard to the reimbursement of GI motility procedures, and inadequate reimbursement should be monitored and periodically addressed by the billing specialists.

Proper coding and billing to get allowable reimbursement is an ongoing learning process and needs to be monitored. When esophageal manometry, pH studies, or endoscopy are performed on the same day, the 51 modifier for multiple procedures on the same day should not be needed because manometry and pH testing are separate diagnostic procedures. A modifier is also not needed when endoscopy and manometry are performed on the same day. This point, however, may have variable responses, depending on the specific payer source. If manometry and prolonged pH studies are performed on day 1, manometry should be billed on day 1 and the pH study should be billed on the day the procedure is terminated. If studies are billed for the same day, it is also best to use separate *International Classification of Diseases, Ninth Revision (ICD-9)* diagnostic codes.

An outline of a method for coding and billing for the esophageal motility laboratory is as follows:

1. Choose the correct procedure code *(CPT)* for the test performed.
2. Chose a clinical diagnosis code *(ICD-9)* that is appropriate for the *CPT* code. The *ICD-9* code should be as specific as possible. Often, the *ICD-9* code is the indication for the test. However, one should try to bill using the appropriate *ICD-9* code for the final, related diagnosis and not for the reason the test was performed. For example, if the esophageal manometry is abnormal, bill for the specific abnormality (eg, 530.0 for achalasia); if the manometry is normal, bill for the indication (eg, 787.1 for heartburn, 787.2 for dysphagia, 786.50 for chest pain).
3. Letters of necessity are occasionally needed to send in with the bill. A template letter of necessity is often valuable.
4. Use electronic software "scrubbers" for reviewing claims and identifying billing or coding errors before submission to insurance company.
5. Monitor the payments and denials.
6. If needed, appeal denials. Have template denial letters for procedures.

Box 6
Billing and coding for the gastrointestinal motility laboratory

Esophageal testing

91010: Esophageal manometry

91011: Esophageal manometry with stimulant (edrophonium)

91012: Esophageal manometry with acid perfusion (Bernstein testing)

91034: Esophageal pH monitoring using nasal catheter pH electrode

91035: Esophageal pH monitoring using mucosal attached telemetry pH probe (Bravo pH system)

91037: Esophageal function testing using gastroesophageal impedance for up to 1 hour

91038: Prolonged gastroesophageal impedance testing for more than 1 hour and up to 24 hours

91040: Esophageal balloon distension provocation testing to evaluate patients who have atypical chest pain

Anorectal testing

91122: Anorectal manometry

90911: Biofeedback training during anal manometry or electromyography

91120: Rectal balloon provocation to measure sensory, motor, and biochemical function of rectum.

45391: Flexible sigmoidoscopy with endoscopic ultrasound

Breath testing

91065: Breath hydrogen testing for lactose intolerance, fructose intolerance, bacterial overgrowth, or evaluation of orocecal transit time

Electrogastrography

91132: Electrogastrography

91133: Electrogastrography with provocative testing (meals, stimulants)

Antroduodenal manometry

91022: Duodenal motility study with the placement of a motility probe into the duodenum

91020: Gastric motility (can both be billed with 91020) if the test is measuring both

If an endoscopy is performed for tube placement, 43235 should be used, and if fluoroscopy is performed, 76000 should be used with 91022

Sphincter of Oddi manometry

43263: Endoscopic retrograde cholangiopancreatography with sphincter of Oddi manometry

Miscellaneous

91299: Unlisted diagnostic gastroenterologic procedure

Note: The 26 modifier is for the professional services component. The technical component modifier is for the technical component.

REGISTRY OF GASTROINTESTINAL MOTILITY LABORATORIES

Proper evaluation of patients who have a possible GI motility disorder is important to provide the proper diagnosis and for the patient to receive optimal care. To provide a meaningful service to physicians and patients, laboratories involved in the conduct of clinical motility studies should meet a set of specified standards that are recognized as appropriate (see **Box 4**). Individuals performing clinical motility studies should be appropriately trained, have sufficient experience in the areas in which they are performing studies, and have appropriate space and equipment to conduct clinical studies. The Clinical Practice Committee of the ANMS has developed a registry of GI motility laboratories that have experience in performing high-quality GI motility procedures commonly used for the evaluation of patients. The purpose of this registry is to have a listing of GI motility laboratories that perform good-quality GI motility testing that can be relied on by other physicians, which will help physicians who want to refer patients, and patients who might need to find a local laboratory that does a particular procedure. The registry also serves several other purposes: (1) identifies GI motility laboratories that perform procedures using appropriate standard methodology; (2) raises awareness of these centers for health care providers who do not have direct access to a GI motility laboratory; (3) raises awareness for patients who are either seeking such centers or wish to be evaluated for their condition. The procedures tracked in the registry are the standard motility procedures, such as esophageal manometry, esophageal pH monitoring, and anorectal manometry. Other procedures tracked include more specialized procedures, such as electrogastrography and antroduodenal manometry. This registry is available at the ANMS website at www.motilitysociety.org.

SUMMARY

Abnormalities of GI motor function contribute directly or indirectly to a number of common clinical problems and account for significant health care–related expenditure.[15] Proper evaluation of patients who have suspected GI motility disorders is important to ensure a correct diagnosis and to embark on an appropriate plan of treatment. The GI motility laboratory serves as an important station for patient evaluation and treatment in gastroenterology and is an essential element in any comprehensive digestive disease program.

ACKNOWLEDGMENTS

The authors would like to acknowledge the suggestions made for this article by Dr. Satish Rao and Dr. Joel Richter.

REFERENCES

1. Drossman DA, Li Z, Andruzzi E, et al. U.S. householder survey of functional gastrointestinal disorders: prevalence, sociodemography, and health impact. Dig Dis Sci 1993;38:1569–80.
2. Russo MW, Wei JT, Thiny MT, et al. Digestive and liver diseases statistics, 2004. Gastroenterology 2004;126:1448–53.
3. Parkman HP, Doma S. The importance of gastrointestinal motility disorders. Pract Gastroenterol 2006;30(9):23–40.
4. Chang L. Epidemiology and quality of life in functional gastrointestinal disorders. Aliment Pharmacol Ther 2004;20(Suppl 7):31–9.
5. Camilleri M, Dubois D, Coulie B, et al. Prevalence and societal impact of upper gastrointestinal disorders in the United States. Clin Gastroenterol Hepatol 2005; 3:543–62.
6. Drossman DA, Corazziari E, Delvaux M, et al, editors. The functional gastrointestinal disorders. 3rd edition. McLean (VA): Degnon Associates; 2006.

7. Galmiche JP, Clouse RE, Balint A, et al. Functional esophageal disorders. Gastroenterology 2006;130:1459–65.

8. AGA Institute Future Trends Committee. Will screening colonoscopy disappear and transform gastroenterology practice? Threats to clinical practice and recommendations to reduce their impact: report of a consensus conference conducted by the AGA Institute Future Trends Committee. Gastroenterology 2006;131: 1287–312.

9. Drossman DA. Manual of gastroenterologic procedures. 2nd edition. New York: Raven Press; 1987.

10. Shaker R, Hofmann C. How to set up and manage a motility laboratory. Goyal & Shaker GI Motility online. Available at: http://www.nature.com/gimo/contents/pt1/full/gimo96.html. Accessed March 25, 2007.

11. Orr WC. Evaluation of laboratory standards for GI motility laboratories. New Wave 2001;1(3). Available at: http://www.giphysiology.org/. Accessed March 25, 2007.

12. Parkman HP. Training in GI motility. Dig Dis 2006;24(3–4):221–7.

13. AASLD, ACG, AGA, et al. Training the gastroenterologists of the future: the gastroenterology core curriculum. Gastroenterology 2003;124:1055–104.

14. Botoman VA, Rao S, Dunlap P, et al. Bill Coding and RVS Committee of the American Motility Society. Motility and GI function studies billing and coding guidelines: a position paper of the American Motility Society. Am J Gastroenterol 2003;98(6):1228–36.

15. Wiley JW, Nostrant TT, Owyang C. Evaluation of gastrointestinal motility: methodologic considerations. In: Yamada T, editor. Textbook of gastroenterology. 4th edition. Philadelphia: Lippincott Williams & Wilkins; 2003. p. 3057–73 [chapter 150].

Index

Note: Page numbers of article titles are in **boldface** type.

A

Aging, as factor in fecal incontinence, 84
Anorectal manometry, in constipation evaluation, 125–126
Anorectal surgery, fecal incontinence associated with, 85
Antegrade colonic edema, 104–105
Antibiotics, intestinal microbiota effects of, clinical data on, 145–146
Antidepressant(s), tricyclic
    for FGIDs, 155–159
    for nausea and vomiting associated with gastroparesis, 67–68
Antiemetics
    classes of, 74
    for nausea and vomiting associated with gastroparesis, 60–65
        cholinergic antagonists, 61–64
        histamine, 61–64
        5-hydroxytryptamine 3 antagonists, 61
        phenothiazines, 60–61
Antipsychotics, atypical, for FGIDs, 161
Antireflux surgery (ARS), for GERD, **35–48**
    care after, 40–41
    outcomes of, 41–42
    patient selection for, 37–38
    principles of, 38–40
    technique of, 38–40
Antroduodenal manometry, in gastric emptying evaluation, 53–54
Artificial bowel sphincter, in fecal incontinence management, 89–90

B

Balloon expulsion test, in constipation evaluation, 126
Barrett's esophagus, treatment of, 43–45
Behavioral therapies, for FGIDs, 152–153, 162–164
    cognitive behavior therapy, 163
    combined psychotherapies, 163
    dynamic interpersonal psychotherapy, 163–164
    general approach to, 162
    hypnotherapy, 164
    limitations of, 164
    mindfulness meditation, 164
    psychopharmacologic therapy with, 165
    relaxation training, 163
Benzodiazepines, for FGIDs, 161
Breath tests, in gastric emptying evaluation, 52
Buspirone, for FGIDs, 161

Gastrointest Endoscopy Clin N Am 19 (2009) 185–192
doi:10.1016/S1052-5157(09)00011-7
1052-5157/09/$ – see front matter © 2009 Elsevier Inc. All rights reserved.

giendo.theclinics.com

Moving?

Make sure your subscription moves with you!

To notify us of your new address, find your **Clinics Account Number** (located on your mailing label above your name), and contact customer service at:

E-mail: elspcs@elsevier.com

800-654-2452 (subscribers in the U.S. & Canada)
314-453-7041 (subscribers outside of the U.S. & Canada)

Fax number: 314-523-5170

Elsevier Periodicals Customer Service
11830 Westline Industrial Drive
St. Louis, MO 63146

*To ensure uninterrupted delivery of your subscription, please notify us at least 4 weeks in advance of move.

Printed and bound by CPI Group (UK) Ltd, Croydon, CR0 4YY

03/10/2024

01040464-0020